Weaning

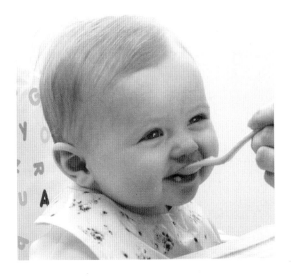

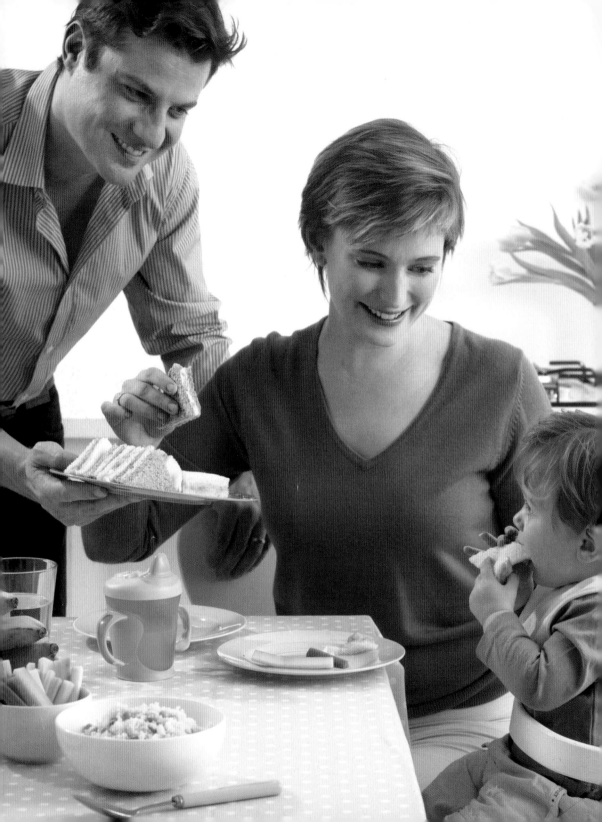

annabel karmel

Weaning

The **essential** guide to baby's **first foods**

Previously published as *Starting Solids*

LONDON • NEW YORK • MUNICH • MELBOURNE • DELHI

I would like to dedicate the book to my
children Nicholas, Lara, and Scarlett

Project editor Helen Murray
Editorial assistance Angela Baynham
US editor Shannon Beatty
US medical consultant Dr. Aviva Schein
Designer Jo Grey
Senior art editor Sara Kimmins
Jacket designer and design assistant Charlotte Seymour
Managing editor Penny Warren
Managing art editors Glenda Fisher and Marianne Markham
Senior production editor Jennifer Murray
Production controller Hema Gohil
Creative technical support Sonia Charbonnier
Category publisher Peggy Vance
Editorial consultant Karen Sullivan
Allergy consultant Dr. Adam Fox
Nutritional consultant Dr. Rosan Meyer
Food styling Seiko Hatfield
Home economist Carolyn Humphries
Photographer Dave King
Photography art direction Peggy Sadler

First American edition, 2010; this edition 2012.
Previously published in 2010 as Starting Solids.

Published in the United States by
DK Publishing
375 Hudson Street
New York, New York 10014

12 13 14 15 16 10 09 08 07 06 05 04 03 02 01
001—175543—September 2012

Published in Great Britain by Dorling Kindersley Limited.

A catalog record for this book is available from the Library of Congress.

ISBN 978-0-7566-9886-7

DK books are available at special discounts when purchased in bulk for
sales promotions, premiums, fund-raising, or educational use. For details,
contact: DK Publishing Special Markets, 375 Hudson Street, New York,
New York 10014 or SpecialSales@dk.com.

Color reproduction by Colourscan, Singapore
Printed and bound in China by Leo

Discover more at
www.dk.com

Contents

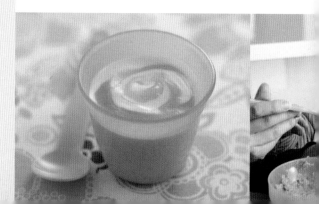

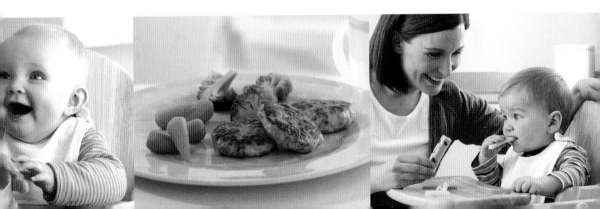

Foreword

Many people have asked me for a book on weaning to help guide them through the first year of their baby's life, from the very first spoonful through to finger foods and family meals. I meet a lot of parents who are confused by conflicting advice from books, websites, doctors, family, and health professionals, and my aim is to help you make your own informed decisions and to give your baby the very best start in life.

I have spent the last 20 years since losing my first child researching and working on improving nutrition and developing recipes for babies and children. I have written 20 books, which have been published all over the world. All my advice is based on scientific research and what I have learned while raising my own three children.

My aim is not just to give parents information on what foods to give and when, but also to help them find ways to make these foods taste delicious—even without added seasoning—so that a baby is trained from an early age to enjoy eating healthy food. Between six months and a year, there is a window of opportunity when babies tend to be pretty good eaters, and it is important to introduce as much variety into the diet as soon as you can so that your child does not grow up to be a fussy eater.

I understand that as a parent of a young baby there isn't the time to be spending hours in the kitchen, so my recipes are quick and easy to prepare. They can also be made in bulk and then frozen in individual portions so, with the help of my menu planners, you can give your baby a good balanced diet while only having to cook a couple of times a week. There are lots of time-saving tips too—for example, how to prepare no-cook baby food by simply mashing banana or avocado. There is also advice on how best to introduce chicken, fish, and meat, and why

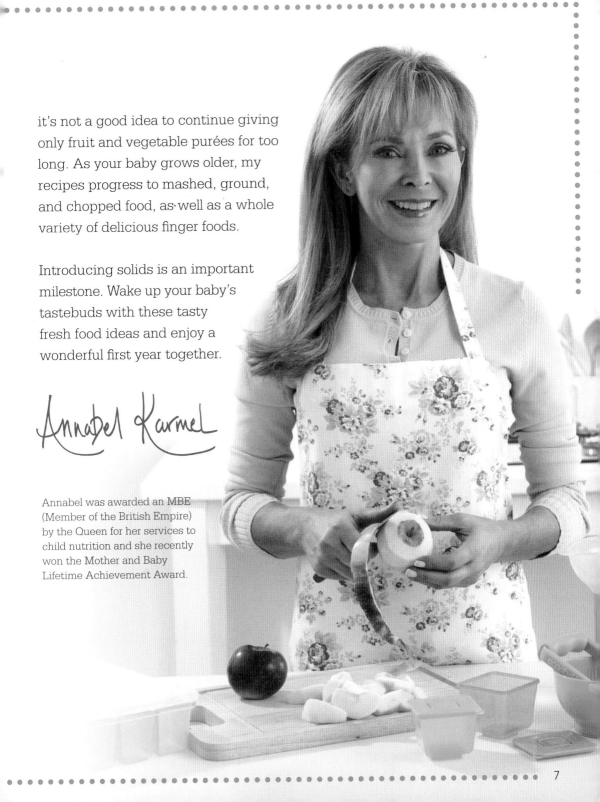

it's not a good idea to continue giving only fruit and vegetable purées for too long. As your baby grows older, my recipes progress to mashed, ground, and chopped food, as well as a whole variety of delicious finger foods.

Introducing solids is an important milestone. Wake up your baby's tastebuds with these tasty fresh food ideas and enjoy a wonderful first year together.

Annabel Karmel

Annabel was awarded an MBE (Member of the British Empire) by the Queen for her services to child nutrition and she recently won the Mother and Baby Lifetime Achievement Award.

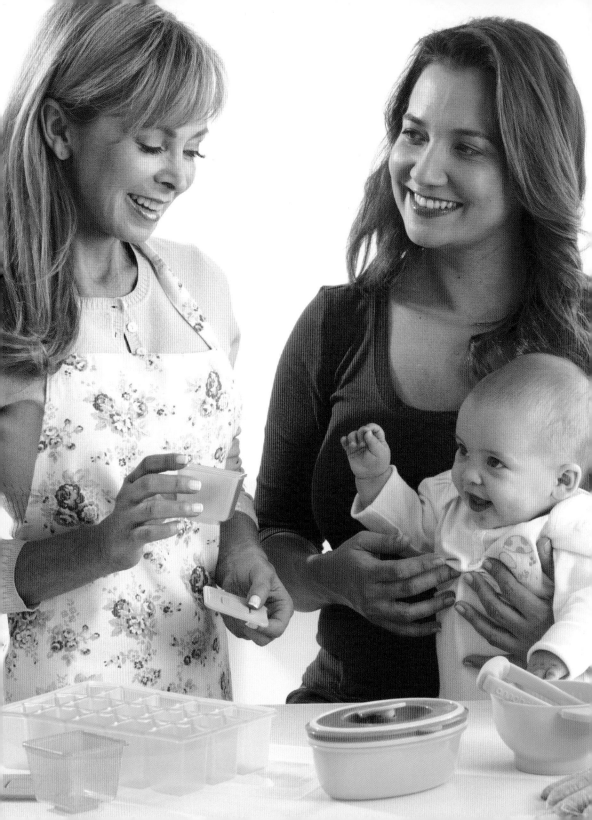

Understanding weaning

The steps involved in **introducing your baby to solid food** are not set in stone and you may find that she progresses more **quickly or more slowly** than other babies of a similar age. **Some days may be better** than others, too, and there will also be times when she wants **only her usual milk.** It helps to understand the basics of weaning and **the theory behind it.** Armed with knowledge, you'll be able to develop a **method that works** for you and your baby.

What weaning's all about

Weaning is a gentle process, involving slowly and sensitively replacing your baby's regular milk with healthy, delicious, nutritious food, which will fill her with energy and encourage optimum growth and development. You have a window of opportunity between 6 and 12 months of age when your baby will tend to eat pretty well, so take advantage of this to introduce a variety of new flavors that will hopefully set her on a path of healthy eating for life.

Your baby's usual milk

From around six months, your baby's regular milk will no longer provide her with all the nutrients she needs—in particular, vitamin D and iron—and her stores of these start becoming depleted by this stage. This is one reason why now is the ideal time to begin weaning, as missing nutrients need to be provided by food. It is, however, very important to remember that your baby's milk will continue to form a significant part of her nutrition for many months to come, giving her the fat, carbohydrates, protein, vitamins, and minerals she needs. What's more, feeding your baby her milk will remain an important source of comfort and will help to continue the bonding process.

Weaning is a gentle process, involving slowly and sensitively replacing your baby's regular milk with healthy, delicious, nutritious food.

Your baby will need breast milk or formula until she is at least 12 months old, when her diet is varied enough to offer the correct balance of nutrients. Breastfeeding can be successfully continued alongside the introduction of solid

Premature babies

Many people think that babies who are born early may be a little late in many stages of development, as they catch up on time lost in the womb. While it is important to monitor your baby's developmental milestones, weaning your little one usually doesn't need to be delayed past six months. Actually, babies born early miss out on some of the normal nourishment that occurs in the womb during the latter stages of pregnancy. In particular, they may need nutrients such as iron and zinc, because these are only stored in the baby's body in the last weeks of pregnancy, and therefore some premature babies need extra nutrition or supplements in order to "catch up." Also, weaning may take them a little longer than full-term babies. If your baby seems ready (see page 22), talk to your doctor. When you begin, go for nutrient-dense foods, such as avocado, potatoes, and apricots, which will help to build her up.

food. There is plenty of research to suggest that breast milk continues to offer antibodies well into toddlerhood, which can help your little one resist infection. It also contains a readily absorbed form of iron, as well as protein, essential fatty acids, vitamins, minerals, and enzymes, making it a perfect complement to a healthy, varied diet.

When starting solids, breastfeed your baby as usual, or, if she is on formula, make sure she gets at least 28oz (840ml) per day. Most parents find it easiest to continue with the morning and evening feeds and fit the other milk feeds around mealtimes, gradually giving a little less as their baby takes more solids. Feed your baby after her first solids instead of before, so that she is hungrier and more willing to try foods being offered. Top her off by filling her tummy with a milk feed once she's had a few spoonfuls of puréed fruit, vegetables, or rice.

Introducing a mixed diet

When you begin to wean your baby, you'll be introducing her to new tastes in the form of baby rice, vegetables, and fruit. At the outset, she'll take these in the form of a liquid purée so that it's similar to her milk—it should be almost the same consistency as yogurt—and then progress to lumpier, thicker purées, then lumps. Variety is the order of the day. Introduce her to a new food every day or so. The greater the variety, the easier it will be to progress to a healthy, nutritious diet. One or more spoonfuls swallowed represents success in the early days, so don't panic if she doesn't manage a whole bowl.

Remember, the first stage of weaning is about introducing new tastes and teaching the art of eating, and it can take some time. So offer each new taste and if she doesn't like what's being offered, put it aside and try again another day.

Tips for starting weaning

Getting it right from the start will make the process of weaning your baby over the coming months much easier. Later on in the book, we'll look at the various setbacks that can arise, and the best ways to deal with them. However, before you even put that first spoonful into your baby's mouth, it's helpful to be aware of the top tips for successful weaning:

✸ Make sure your baby is ready. Pushing a young, reluctant baby will make the start of the weaning process upsetting for you both (see page 22).

✸ Babies sometimes find the process a little clinical and become upset when mealtimes no longer involve the comfort of sucking milk. When offering your baby her very first taste or two you may find it easier to hold her on your lap, as this will help her feel loved and secure.

✸ When babies feed from the breast or a bottle they instinctively push their tongue forward. Now your baby needs to learn to keep her tongue at the back of her mouth. If she has trouble with a spoon, try dipping a clean finger in the purée and let her suck your finger for the first few mouthfuls.

✸ Laugh, smile, sing, and taste your baby's food at mealtimes—she'll want to join in the fun by copying you and eating it herself.

✸ Avoid feeding your baby when she's tired, irritable, or very hungry. At these times, she'll want one thing only—milk.

✸ Don't get too hung up about portion sizes or nutrients. If the food is wholesome and fresh and she's eating a little, you've done well.

✸ Try not to compare your baby with others. All babies develop at their own speed and take to different foods at different stages. It is no reflection on their intelligence or abilities.

Weaning truths and myths

The process of weaning is surrounded by myths. We've got grandma telling us that babies need to be weaned at three or four months in order to sleep through the night, then reports suggesting we're giving babies a lifetime of health problems if we do it sooner than six months. So what is the truth?

Sleeping through

Many babies continue to wake up at night, which can be exhausting for parents. If this is the case with your little one, once the weaning process is underway make sure you give him a nutritious evening meal that contains a carbohydrate, a protein, and a vegetable (see page 16). Protein in particular takes a long time to digest and may help to keep your child satisfied for a longer period of time if he is waking up due to hunger.

Teething and weaning

The development of teeth doesn't mean your baby is ready for solids. Some babies cut their first milk teeth around four months, which is early for weaning, while others show no signs of teething until well after six months.

Weight gain

It's often suggested that underweight babies benefit from early weaning; however, research shows that continuing with milk feeds encourages your baby to reach his optimum weight as initial foods (fruit and vegetables) are often low in energy.

Late weaning and allergies

Some parents have been advised to wean their babies later than six months because of a family history of allergies. The idea is that their immune systems would be more mature later on and better able to cope with allergens. In fact,

research has found that later weaning has no impact on the development of allergies but may make it more difficult to encourage your baby to eat solid foods. What's more, he runs the risk of becoming iron deficient, as his regular milk will not contain enough to meet his needs. Weaning at around six months is ideal.

Avoiding wheat, meat, and dairy

Some parents decide to keep their babies' diets clear of wheat, meat, and dairy. However, cutting out whole food groups is dangerous. Dairy is an important source of calcium and vitamin D—vital for teeth and bone growth. It's also a good source of protein. Wheat is a source of gluten, which can cause problems in a minority of babies; however, it is also a great source of carbohydrates, B vitamins, and fiber. After six months, it's a healthy addition to your baby's diet. As for meat, there are few other such readily available sources of easily absorbed iron.

Odd bowel movements

If foods reappear undigested in your baby's diaper, you may think he's not ready for weaning. Be assured that many foods seem untouched by the digestive process, but some goodness will have been absorbed. Until they are about two, babies cannot completely digest husked vegetables and fruit skins. Peeling, mashing, and puréeing encourages foods to be digested.

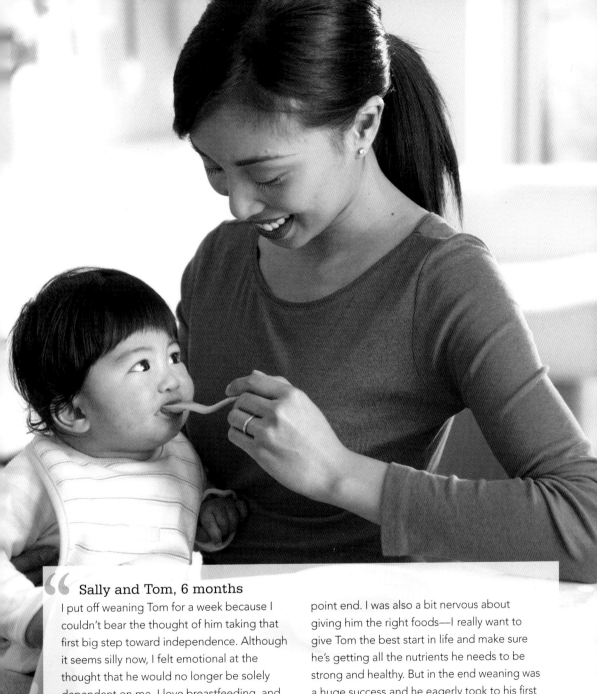

Sally and Tom, 6 months

I put off weaning Tom for a week because I couldn't bear the thought of him taking that first big step toward independence. Although it seems silly now, I felt emotional at the thought that he would no longer be solely dependent on me. I love breastfeeding, and we both found it hugely comforting. Solid food seemed so clinical and it was a big reminder that our lovely feeds would at some point end. I was also a bit nervous about giving him the right foods—I really want to give Tom the best start in life and make sure he's getting all the nutrients he needs to be strong and healthy. But in the end weaning was a huge success and he eagerly took to his first tastes. For our first purée, I chose organic sweet potatoes with a little expressed breast milk. At least I know he's getting the best there is!

Creating a healthy diet

Everything your baby eats contributes to her growth and development, and lays the foundation for her future health. While the process of weaning is initially more about an introduction to the world of food than a prescription for good health, little spoonfuls lead to bigger ones, and it's important to introduce variety to help prevent your baby from becoming a fussy eater.

You don't have to be an expert in nutrition to create healthy, nutritious meals for your baby. Choosing fresh, unprocessed foods will boost her health and make sure that she gets all the nutrients she requires.

So what does your baby need? From birth until around six months, she'll get everything she needs from her regular milk, whether breast or bottle. Breastfeeding is the healthiest option (see page 11), and you can continue with this for as long as you both feel happy, alongside other foods. However, the fact that your baby is getting most of her nutrients from milk doesn't mean that you can skimp on the quality of other foods.

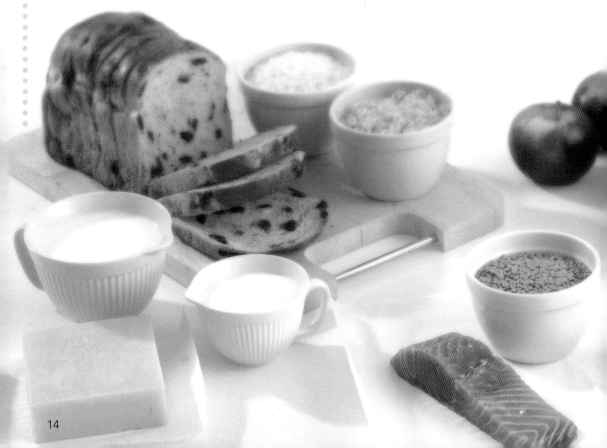

A balanced diet simply means a diet that contains all of the elements that contribute to good health. This is what it should contain:

Fats

We've been conditioned to think that fat is "unhealthy," but this simply isn't the case. It's actually important for energy and all sorts of body functions, including the nervous system. Fats contain vitamins A, D, and E, which are also crucial for health and development.

The most important type of fats are "essential fatty acids," or EFAs, which you can find in oily fish, nuts, seeds, vegetable oils, and avocados. These play a key role in your baby's brain and visual development in the first year, and it's important to introduce fish such as salmon into her diet once the first tastes (see Chapter 2) are established.

The fats to avoid are transfats, which have been hydrogenated. They have been shown to have an adverse health effect and are used in all kinds of processed and baked food, including cookies, pies, potato chips, and cakes. Avoid anything with the word "hydrogenated" on the label.

Saturated fats, such as those found in cheese, butter, whole milk, and meat, have also been linked with health problems; however, babies do need proportionately more of these fats in their diet than adults due to their fast growth rate, so it's a good idea to add a little cheese or butter to your baby's purée once the initial feeding stage (see Chapter 2) is established.

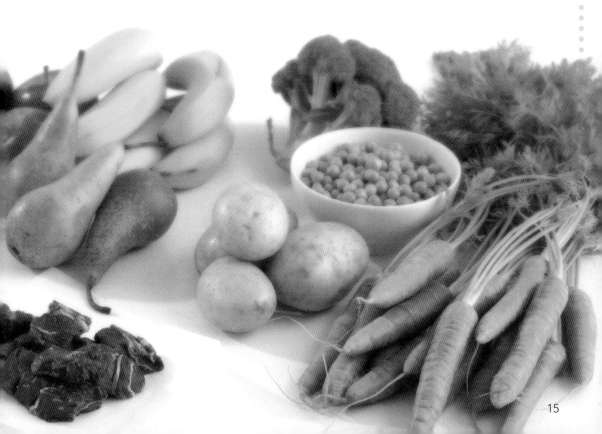

Carbohydrates

Foods that contain carbohydrates are considered to be "energy" foods and will provide your baby with most of her "fuel." Complex carbohydrates, which are those that are unrefined, such as wholegrain cereals and breads, brown rice, fruit, and vegetables, are the healthiest. However, these also provide fiber. It is not good for babies to have too much fiber, though, because this fills them up very quickly and reduces the absorption of essential vitamins and minerals. Refined carbs, such as white rice and flour, have a slightly lower nutritional value, but they make better starter foods for babies because they are more easily digestible. As she becomes older, your baby will move from refined cereals and baby rice to more complex carbohydrates.

Proteins

Protein is found in fish, lean meats, poultry, legumes (such as chickpeas, beans, and lentils), soy, dairy products, and eggs. It gives your baby the building blocks for good, steady growth and healthy development and is an essential part of her diet. If you've chosen to give your baby a vegan or vegetarian diet, you'll need to make sure that she gets enough good-quality protein (see page 18), as animal sources tend to be the most easily digested and absorbed.

Fiber

This isn't a nutrient as such, but it does have an important role to play in your baby's body. Chewing fiber-rich foods stimulates saliva, which protects your baby's teeth (when they appear), and encourages healthy digestion. It clears out the digestive tract, encourages regular, healthy bowel movements, and helps make sure that the nutrients in your baby's food are efficiently

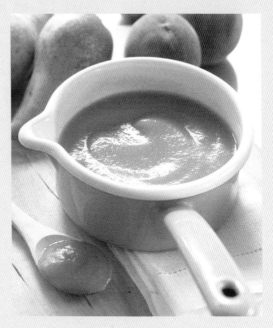

Peach, apple, and pear. Fruit purées are a great source of the vitamins and minerals your baby needs after six months.

absorbed. Pectin, which is a soluble fiber found in apples and carrots, helps to balance blood sugar and encourage healthy immunity. Fiber is found in almost all fruit, vegetables, and grains.

Vitamins and minerals

A balanced diet with plenty of healthy fat, good-quality protein, complex carbohydrates, and fresh vegetables and fruit will contain all the nutrients your baby needs. There are, however, a few others to watch out for:

✹ Iron is extremely important for little ones, and a deficiency can mean your baby is less physically active and may develop more slowly. Not having enough iron can lead to problems concentrating and a shorter attention span, and can leave your baby feeling tired and weak. There are two main types of iron—heme and nonheme. Heme iron is found in meats, fish, and eggs, and is more easily absorbed by your child's body. Nonheme iron comes from plant sources such as legumes, leafy green vegetables, peas, and wholegrains, or iron-fortified cereals. The best advice is to offer a mix of both.

★ Vitamin C is essential for iron absorption, so try to include plenty of fresh fruits and vegetables in your baby's diet. Vitamin C also helps to encourage healthy immune function, healing, and healthy bones and skin. Good sources are fresh fruit and vegetables.

★ Vitamin D is crucial for healthy bones and teeth. Our bodies can manufacture vitamin D if we get enough natural sunlight, and it is also found in dairy products, eggs, oily fish, and fish oil. Breastfed infants over the age of six months and those who consume less than 16oz (500ml) of formula per day should be given a multivitamin supplement that contains a good quantity of vitamin D.

★ Calcium is essential for the growth and development of strong bones and teeth and has a wide range of other functions in your baby's body. Breast milk is naturally high in calcium, and formula also contains good levels to maintain calcium stores. You'll find calcium in dairy products, leafy green vegetables, canned salmon and sardines, sesame seeds, almonds, and soy.

★ Zinc is essential for the proper development of your baby. It is needed for wound-healing, immunity, healthy growth, energy, and normal appetite. You can find zinc in seafood, poultry, lean red meats, sunflower seeds, peanuts, wholegrains, and legumes.

There are other vitamins and minerals that are also required by babies for good health and development, and we'll be looking at these throughout the book.

First tastes

Your baby's first tastes are not intended to provide every known nutrient; however, because babies have small tummies, everything you serve should go some way toward helping her become strong and healthy. Babies also have fewer nutrient stores to draw from, which means that a balanced nutritional intake is important. What's more, likes and dislikes are established early, so helping your baby to develop a taste for healthy foods now will make mealtimes a lot easier in years to come.

When you first introduce your baby to solid foods, portion sizes aren't important. A few spoonfuls, once a day, will give her a taste of different flavors and provide a little nutrition. After a few weeks, your baby will probably begin to eat one or two "meals" a day. "Meals" can, however, be comprised of just a spoonful or two.

You'll find your baby will let you know how much she needs to eat; some foods, such as carbohydrates, will fill her more quickly than fresh fruit and vegetables. When she appears to be full, or resists your attempts to feed her, it's a good idea to stop.

By the time your baby is on three meals a day and cutting down on her milk feeds (around 10 months) she needs to to be eating plenty of fresh fruits and vegetables, good sources of protein, healthy fats, and good-quality carbohydrates to keep her diet balanced, her body healthy, and her energy levels high. Look at her diet throughout the day—as long as she is getting a little of each (ideally some carbohydrate, protein, and vegetable or fruit at every meal), you are doing well.

Special diets

Whether you've chosen to remove certain foods from your baby's diet on health, religious, environmental, or ethical grounds, or his diet has to be restricted for other reasons, it's important to make sure that you make up for any shortfalls to guarantee he's getting all the nutrients he needs.

Vegetarian babies

The good news is that for the first 12 months of your baby's life, he will get most of the vitamins, minerals, and other nutrients he needs from his regular milk. Most babies start off vegetarian anyway, as fruit and vegetable purées form the basis of their diets for the first month or so of weaning. After this initial stage, when you would normally go on to introduce meat, poultry, and fish, you will need to look for alternative sources of iron, protein, zinc, and vitamin B_{12} for your vegetarian baby. Vitamin B_{12} is needed for healthy red blood cells, your baby's nervous system, and healthy growth and development and you can find it in eggs and dairy products. A shortfall can lead to anemia.

Offering dairy products, legumes such as lentils, fortified cereals, and other grains including soy products, leafy green vegetables, and fruit (including dried fruit), should help make sure your baby gets the nutrients that he needs. Provided there is no family history of allergy (see page 20), you can introduce peanut butter at this stage too. You'll also need to make sure that your baby is getting enough EFAs (see page 15)—plant-based sources of healthy fat that include avocado, nut butters, quinoa, olive oil, and flaxseed oil.

Be aware that a vegetarian diet tends to be high in fiber, which is unsuitable for babies. It can also hinder iron absorption and is low in calories as well as essential fats. If your baby is being brought up on a vegetarian diet, it's important to include cheese and well-cooked eggs once initial weaning is established, as these are both nutrient-dense foods.

Vegan babies

Once again, your baby will get the majority of nutrients he needs from his regular milk. However, once he is eating a full diet, you'll need to look for alternative sources of protein, zinc, calcium, vitamin B_{12} (see above), and vitamin D (mainly found in eggs, oily fish, and legumes). Your baby will most likely need a vitamin D supplement and perhaps multivitamin and mineral drops to make up for deficiencies.

It's particularly important to make sure that he is getting some iron from the outset, so look for iron-fortified cereals and include dried fruits, particularly apricots (dried or fresh), and plenty of leafy green vegetables in your purées. Iron in non-meat sources is difficult for us to absorb, so give your baby some vitamin C-rich foods (fruit, vegetables, a small amount of juice) at the same meal to boost iron absorption.

Vitamins and other supplements

Until the age of 12 months, most babies get the nutrients they require from their regular milk. At six months, however, your baby's iron stores start to become depleted and breast milk does not provide sufficient amounts, so it is important to get your little one screened for iron deficiency anemia and progress with weaning foods that contain iron, such as fortified cereal and meat.

Feeding a sick baby

The best advice when your little one is sick is to follow your instincts: if your baby is hungry, offer him something to eat. If he does show an interest in food, stick to baby rice, ripe bananas, and apples—these place no pressure on the digestive system, but offer a little nutrition and energy. If he is not interested in solids, continue offering his usual milk feeds—the most important thing is to keep him hydrated. Bottle-fed babies may require a little extra water, too. If he is off his milk, seek advice from your doctor, who may recommend an oral rehydration solution. Most illnesses shift within 24 to 48 hours, but if your baby seems listless and has few wet diapers (signs of dehydration), see your doctor immediately.

Weight worries

Breastfeeding is the most effective way to prevent a baby from becoming overweight, and breastfed babies are much less likely to develop problems with obesity in later life. If you are bottlefeeding, watch how and when you feed your baby. Look for cues that he is full, and then stop. Babies less than six months don't usually need more than 32oz (960ml) of milk per day. Similarly, when you start introducing solids, try to avoid over-feeding him—offer tastes, and when he loses interest, stop.

If your little one is underweight, make sure he's getting enough of his usual milk and allow him to eat as much as he likes. Make sure that every meal has a source of protein, and you can include healthy fats such as egg, milk, cream, cheese, soy, and olive oil by stirring them into his purées.

Jenny asks . . .

We plan to bring up our baby daughter as a vegetarian, but she doesn't seem to have much energy and I'm worried that her limited diet might be making her ill.

The most important thing to consider is your baby's iron intake. Iron is found in high levels in fortified cereals, legumes, leafy green vegetables, and dried fruit, such as apricots. However, it is most easily absorbed from animal sources such as red meat, although you can improve absorption from non-animal sources by including some vitamin C at mealtimes. This means adding fresh fruit or diluted fruit juice, preferably after your baby's meal (so she isn't too full). You'll also want to be sure she is getting enough carbohydrates, which are the fuel your baby needs for growth and energy. Include some pasta, oats, rice, potatoes, avocados, and refined grains at mealtimes, alongside her vegetables. If nothing seems to make a difference, talk to your doctor, who may check her iron level and prescribe a supplement if it is low.

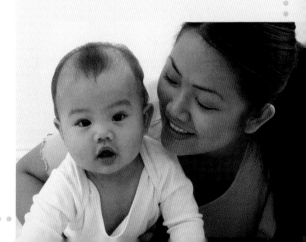

Allergy concerns

Childhood food allergies seem to be on the increase, so it's not surprising that parents are nervous about introducing foods that could cause problems. Assessing whether your baby may be at risk, and learning to recognize the signs of food allergies, can help make weaning safe and successful.

What are allergies?

Allergies occur when your baby's immune system becomes confused. Instead of ignoring harmless food proteins, they trigger a reaction that causes a chemical called histamine to be released. This is responsible for the symptoms associated with allergies, such as hives, skin rashes, and swelling. Reactions can be more severe, causing anaphylaxis, which can be life-threatening.

Most serious food allergies start in infancy and the preschool years and are often outgrown. The same few foods seem to be the culprits in most cases, although these foods vary according to where you live. For example, milk and egg allergies are common worldwide, whereas peanut and tree-nut allergies tend to be most problematic in the US, UK, and Australia, and fish is a common allergen in Spain and Japan. This reflects cultural dietary habits. The most common allergens are eggs, dairy products, wheat, soy, nuts, sesame seeds, fish, peanuts, and shellfish.

Babies at risk

If you have a family history of allergic conditions, such as hay fever, asthma, or eczema, your baby will be at increased risk. Babies who suffer from eczema are more likely to suffer from food allergies. If this is the case, you will need to be more cautious when introducing new foods and wait a little longer between each to see if there is a reaction.

There is no evidence that weaning later or avoiding introducing potentially allergic foods (including peanuts) will affect the likelihood of developing allergies. In fact, feeding your baby a wide variety of foods between six and 12 months can help prevent allergies from developing in later life. What's more, exclusive breastfeeding for six months may also help to prevent allergies in susceptible babies.

When to be worried

The most important thing you can do is to introduce foods to your baby one by one, and wait at least 24 hours between trying new foods. If your baby is in the "at risk" category, wait 48 to 72 hours. Some food allergies are very easy to

Anaphylaxis

All food allergies are potentially dangerous, but if your baby has symptoms that affect her breathing, call an ambulance immediately. This is an anaphylactic reaction, which can cause a drop in blood pressure known as "shock." Symptoms include breathing problems, sudden pallor, inexplicable and sudden drowsiness, facial swelling, and even collapse.

spot (known as "immediate" allergies). A rash may develop around your baby's mouth, her lips, eyes, and face may swell, and her nose may run. She may also vomit or have diarrhea. If her breathing is affected, it's vital you call an ambulance immediately, as this is a life-threatening reaction. The same applies if your baby suddenly looks pale or if she loses consciousness.

Some allergies can be delayed and this makes them harder to detect. Symptoms can include eczema, reflux, poor growth, constipation or diarrhea, tummy pain, and frequent distress or crying. However, many of these symptoms commonly occur in childhood and allergies may be only one explanation. For this reason it is important to see an experienced doctor to decide whether food is at the root of the problem.

" Most serious food allergies start in infancy and the preschool years and are often outgrown. "

Food intolerance

Intolerance is different than a food allergy, because it does not involve the immune system. Instead, some cases involve a shortage of enzymes, which makes digesting the problem food difficult. For example, in the case of lactose intolerance, there is a shortage of the enzyme lactase, which is involved in the digestion of milk. Some intolerance is temporary. Your baby may develop a short-term intolerance to milk after a tummy bug, for example. Very rarely, your baby can experience an intolerance to the chemicals added to foods, such as colorings, flavorings, monosodium glutamate (MSG), and sulphites. Symptoms can be similar to those of a food

allergy, and it can be difficult to distinguish between them. If your baby is suffering from any unusual symptoms after eating particular foods, it's important that you take her to see your doctor.

Keeping a food journal

One of the best ways to pinpoint problem foods is to make a note of what your baby eats. Jot down every food you introduce, when you introduce it, and any reactions your baby may have to it. Even if your baby doesn't suffer from allergies, it can be useful to record details of what foods she has tried and what you think she thought of them! If you do have allergies in the family, it is advisable to wait 48 hours between the introduction of potentially allergenic foods to see if there is a reaction. So, try dairy products, for example, and then wait for two days before introducing eggs on the third day.

It is a good idea to introduce new foods at breakfast or lunchtime, so you can monitor your baby's reaction throughout the remainder of the day. Continue to make a note of any changes in your baby's health and even in her sleep patterns, bowel movements, and behavior for a few days after the introduction of any new food.

What if there is a reaction?

If you do notice a reaction, then stop feeding your baby the new food in question, and make an appointment to see your doctor, who can arrange for your baby to see an allergy specialist. The best treatment for a food allergy is to avoid the problem food completely. This may mean you will need to make up for any nutritional shortfalls by giving other foods, but your doctor can arrange for you to see a dietitian, who can provide specialist help. Many food allergies are outgrown in childhood.

Is your baby ready for weaning?

A great deal of emphasis has been placed on weaning babies at the "right" time and there are good grounds for this. However, before you embark on those first tastes of solid food, it is equally important that your baby is ready.

Exclusive breastfeeding for the first six months of your baby's life is suggested for a variety of reasons. Breast milk is a complete food for babies, providing them with nutrients as well as liquid to keep them hydrated. Your breast milk also provides additional benefits, such as antibodies against infections, hormones, EFAs, enzymes, and living cells. That said, introducing your baby to solids is about offering new tastes. Some babies are ready earlier than others, although solids should not be given before 17 weeks.

The four- to six-month window

From 17 weeks onward, many babies can tolerate some solids and it's important to introduce solid food by 24 weeks. Here's why:

✸ Your baby has the digestive enzymes required.
✸ He has some head control and can maintain a good position for swallowing.

Coping with allergies

It is suggested that babies who have a family history of allergies will benefit from exclusive breastfeeding for six months before starting on solids. After this, you can wean as usual, paying particular attention to potentially allergenic foods (see pages 20–21).

✸ His kidneys can cope with solid foods.
✸ His iron reserves begin to deplete around six months and it becomes increasingly important that he gets some iron from his diet. Iron is an important factor in brain development.
✸ His jaw and tongue have developed to cope with eating and swallowing foods.
✸ Dealing with solid foods helps your baby's mouth and tongue develop and prepare for speaking.
✸ Up to six months, babies readily accept new tastes, flavors, and textures. If you wait too long, your baby may become more resistant. Breastfed babies will be used to a variety of flavors through their mother's milk and may take to new foods more easily than bottle-fed babies.

Signs your baby is ready

Your baby will start to show some interest in what you are eating and perhaps reach out to taste it. He may be hungrier than usual, often unsatisfied after his normal milk feed, and possibly waking in the night, when he previously slept through.

It's worth noting that a growth spurt commonly occurs between three and four months, which may cause him to wake more at night and perhaps feed more frequently, so don't assume at this age that he's ready for solids just yet.

Other signs that he is ready, include:
✸ Holding his head up; controlling movements.
✸ Attempting to put things into his mouth.
✸ Making chewing motions.
✸ Chewing on his fingers or fists.

Offering new foods

Below is a guide to the foods that are appropriate for your baby's growth and development at each stage of weaning—bear in mind that some babies are ready for a greater variety of new foods earlier than others.

⭐ Stage One – around 6 months	⭐ Stage Two – 6 to 9 months	⭐ Stage Three – 10 to 12 months
Consistency Semi-liquid purées; easy-to-gum finger foods, depending on your baby's ability to gum and chew (see page 44)	Thicker purées, adding tiny lumps and mashed or finely ground food; melt-in-the-mouth and bite-and-dissolve finger foods (see pages 70–71)	Ground, chopped, mashed, and lumpy food; bite-and-chew finger foods (see pages 70–71)
Fruits Ripe peaches, bananas, apples, pears, papaya, mango, melon, avocado	Plums, nectarines, berries, cherries, dried apricots, guava	Citrus fruit (but watch for a reaction); other dried fruit; continue to expand your baby's repertoire of fruit
Vegetables Potatoes, rutabaga, carrots, parsnips, sweet potatoes, butternut squash, pumpkin	Corn, spinach, peas, cauliflower, zucchini, broccoli, green beans, onions, sweet peppers, mushrooms	Continue to expand your baby's repertoire of vegetables (e.g., sugar snap peas and baby sweetcorn)
Cereals and grains Gluten-free cereals such as baby rice, millet, and quinoa	Any grains, such as rice, barley, oats, wheat in bread, pasta, breakfast cereals, couscous	Continue to expand your baby's repertoire of grains, including brown rice, whole grains, and flaxseeds
	Protein Chicken, white and oily fish, well-cooked eggs, red meat, tofu, legumes, nut butters, very finely ground nuts	Continue to expand your baby's repertoire of proteins, including different cuts of meat and new varieties of fish
	Dairy products Hard pasteurized cheeses, cottage and cream cheese, full-fat plain yogurt, cow's milk (in cooking and with cereal), butter	Soft pasteurized cheeses

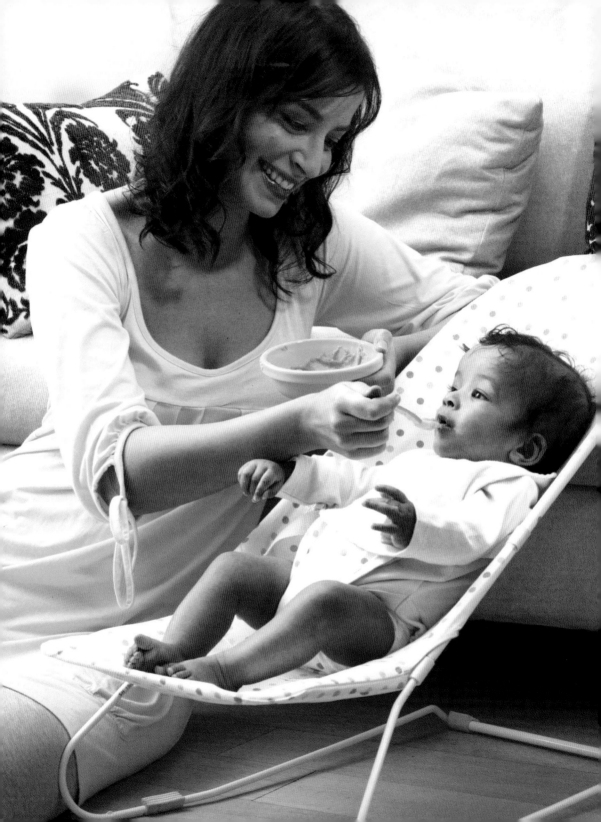

stage one – around 6 months

First tastes

Your baby's first tastes **mark a big milestone in her life** and can be both exhilarating and nerve-racking for you. Preparing equipment and ingredients in advance **and getting acquainted** with the best first foods can help make the process easier. The **best advice** is to take it slowly, spend time planning your baby's meals, and **go at her pace.** She'll soon get into the swing of things and enjoy **experimenting** with a variety of different tastes.

✱ Menu planners pages 56–57

Getting started: what you'll need

A little planning makes weaning your baby that much easier and you'll be surprised how little equipment you need to prepare nutritious, delicious first foods. You may already have most things you need to get started, and buying a few carefully chosen items will help to make mealtimes an enjoyable and positive experience for you and your baby.

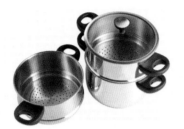
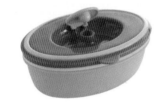

☆ A steamer

Not only does this provide a quick and easy way to cook fruit, vegetables, fish, and poultry, but steaming also helps preserve essential nutrients, making sure your baby gets the most from what she eats.

☆ A microwave steamer

This is a small pot with a valve in the lid that allows steam to escape. Steaming in the microwave is an excellent way to cook small portions of fruit, vegetables, and fish quickly and efficiently, while maintaining their nutritional value.

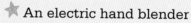

★ An electric hand blender

This is great for making small quantities of baby food, and for puréeing family meals for your baby (you can freeze these in small portions and use them as you need them). A hand blender is essential if you don't have a food processor. Look out for a model that has several speeds.

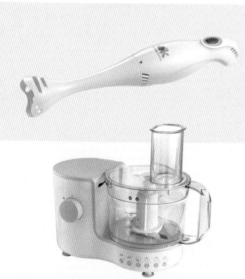

★ A food processor

This is ideal for producing larger quantities of purées for freezing, and some also come with mini bowl attachments for whipping up small quantities when required. Choose a food processor with a variety of blades for creating textured foods later on.

Key	★ Essential	☆ Useful

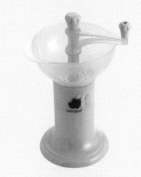

☆ A mouli (small food grinder)

A mouli is ideal for foods with tougher skins, such as peas or dried fruit, making it easier to separate the less digestible parts. It is also the best way to purée a potato (using a food processor makes it get sticky).

★ A masher

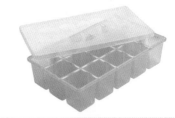

A potato-masher, or even a potato ricer (sort of like a large garlic press), is perfect for creating lumpier textures. Look for a mini-masher, making it easy to mash and crush small amounts of food.

★ An ice-cube tray

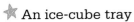

Freeze small portions of purée in ice-cube trays and pop out a portion or two to defrost as required. Choose a flexible tray with a lid. Perhaps consider buying several trays in different colors, which may help you identify the contents.

★ A thermos

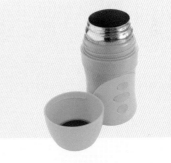

A wide-necked thermos, which will keep food warm or cool for several hours, is ideal for transporting food for your baby. This can also be used to carry hot water, which can then be used for warming baby food. Look for a thermos that can be used in the microwave and washed in the dishwasher.

★ A bib

Babies are messy, no matter how careful you are. Plastic wipe-clean bibs are useful, as well as those with a curve at the base to collect food that doesn't make it to her mouth. Choose a bib that fits comfortably under your baby's chin. Younger babies may prefer soft, cotton ones.

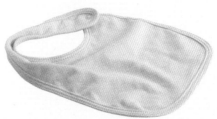

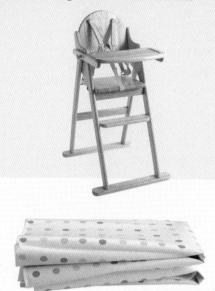

⭐ A high chair

Choose a chair that will wipe clean easily. Small babies require a padded insert for support and a five-point harness is essential. High chairs that can be raised or lowered to allow sitting at the table are also useful. If your baby isn't ready for a high chair, his car seat or baby seat is fine.

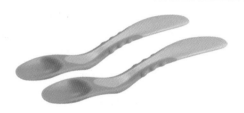

☆ A mess mat

Placed under your baby's chair, this mat will protect carpets and flooring from inevitable spills. Choose one that is non-slip, stain-resistant, and wipe-clean. Large mats are ideal, as your baby's firing range will undoubtedly increase as he gets older.

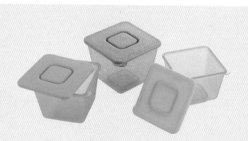

⭐ Feeding spoons

Choose a soft, plastic spoon that won't hurt your baby's gums. It should be small enough to fit easily into his mouth and have a long handle. It's never too soon to get babies used to holding a spoon and giving self-feeding a try (see page 39).

⭐ Small bowls

To begin with, you'll need small food containers that you can hold in one hand—these are ideal for freezing, storing, and reheating food, and you can also feed your baby from them (see page 39). Choose ones with lids to make transportation easy, and make sure they are dishwasher safe.

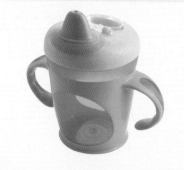

⭐ A lidded cup

From six months, milk and other drinks should be offered in a cup. Avoid the non-spill type as these require your baby to continue sucking rather than learning to drink. The liquid should flow freely, but not too quickly. Some brands have specific flow settings, which can be set according to your baby's age. Soft, easy-to-grip handles are essential.

Which foods should I choose?

Your baby's food should be as fresh as possible, without any added ingredients, such as colorings, flavorings, salt, or sugar. Choosing fresh or frozen local produce will help you make sure he gets the nutrients he needs.

Fresh or frozen?

While fresh food would appear to be healthier for your baby, the truth is that a good proportion of the produce we eat has been picked well before its prime and has probably then sat in the back of a truck or on a supermarket shelf for some time. If you can get fresh food from your supermarket with a quick turnover or a farmers' market (or, indeed, grow it yourself), fresh is best. However, second best is most definitely frozen. Frozen food has been flash-frozen, often minutes after picking, and it maintains the highest level of nutrients.

Local and seasonal

Locally grown food spends less time being packaged and transported, and therefore contains a higher number of nutrients. Organic co-ops and farmers' markets are good sources, or you can grow your own. Most locally grown food will also be in season. Fruit and vegetables in season are less expensive, and also likely to be fresher and more nutritious.

Raw or cooked?

Ideally, raw fruits and vegetables contain a greater quantity as well as different types of nutrients than cooked. More than half the nutrients of raw foods are destroyed in the cooking process, depending on the way you cook them (see page 34). Raw foods contain enzymes that are required by the body to break down other foods, which helps us to absorb what we need from what we eat. Having

said that, raw foods tend to be high in fiber, which is not ideal for little tummies. What's more, research shows that we absorb more nutrients from some cooked foods than we would if they were raw. Carrots and tomatoes are good examples. What's the answer? A few soft, raw, fresh foods (mangoes and bananas) make delicious and nutritious purées for babies. However, until weaning is established and they are eating regular meals, the majority of their food should be cooked.

Going organic?

Although organic food, which is grown and processed without the use of artificial chemicals and potentially dangerous pesticides, has been proven to be better for the environment, there is little evidence to support claims that it is more nutritious. That said, some parents who make their own purées using organic ingredients believe that they have more natural sweetness and flavor, which helps when introducing babies to food. Be aware, however, that because of strict guidelines governing what can and can't be added to organic products, you won't find foods fortified with iron and calcium, which is important for growing babies.

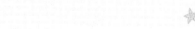

best first vegetables . . . . . carrot

Best first foods

A plain purée of a single root vegetable mixed with your baby's usual milk is the perfect first food. Your baby will be used to the sweet taste of milk, so choose sweet vegetables to start.

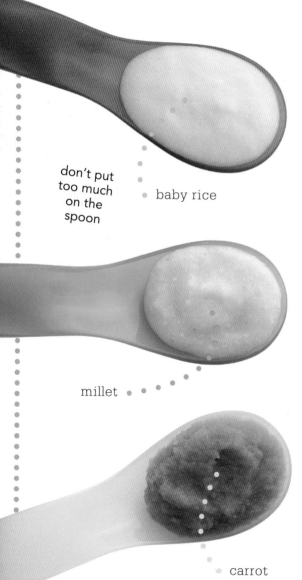

don't put too much on the spoon

baby rice

millet

carrot

It's fine to start with single fruit purées, too, although it's best to follow vegetable purées with fruit, as some babies may figure out that the fruit is sweeter, and may reject the vegetables.

Baby rice

Mixed with water, breast milk, or formula, baby rice has a sweet, milky taste and is easily digested. It can be blended to almost any consistency, making it an ideal starter food. Choose a brand that is sugar-free and enriched with vitamins and iron and follow the instructions on the package. Avoid gluten-containing cereals, such as wheat, rye, and barley, until your baby is at least six months old.

Millet

This gluten-free cereal is a good starter food for little ones and has a mild, sweet, nut-like flavor. It contains B vitamins, some vitamin E, and is particularly high in iron, which is important for growing babies. Millet blends well with your baby's usual milk and both fruits and vegetables. Simply follow the instructions on the packet.

Carrot

The sweet taste of carrots appeals to babies. Cook them until they are soft enough to purée (see page 46). Orange-colored root vegetables are rich in beta-carotene, which is essential for your baby's growth, healthy skin, good vision, and strong bones.

potato pumpkin sweet potato

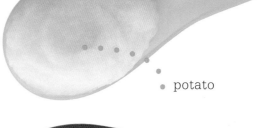

potato

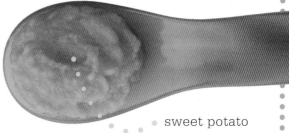

sweet potato

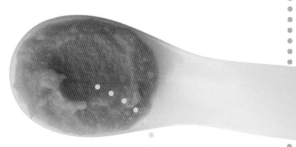

Potato

Mild-tasting and a good source of vitamin C and potassium, potatoes make a great first weaning food. Peel and chop, then put into a pan, cover with boiling water, and cook for 15 minutes or until tender. Alternatively, steam until tender. Use a mouli or food grinder to purée, as an electric blender breaks down the starches and produces a sticky pulp. You can also bake the potato in the oven for 1–1¼ hours, scoop out the flesh, and mash with a little of your baby's usual milk.

Sweet potato

Packed with beta-carotene, sweet potato (see page 48) is richer in nutrients than ordinary potatoes. What's more, almost any vegetable when combined with sweet potatoes will taste delicious.

Butternut squash

Another colorful vegetable rich in beta-carotene, butternut squash (see page 47) has a smooth, mild flavor. Try combining it with apple and pear, or keep it simple and just mix with a little baby rice.

butternut squash

colorful food equals plenty of nutrients

Pumpkin

The orange flesh of this vegetable is sweet and bursting with vitamin C and beta-carotene. Peel and chop, then boil or steam, or bake wedges in the oven (see page 47). Pumpkin purées to a smooth consistency and combines well with fruit, other vegetables, and baby rice, making it a popular early weaning food.

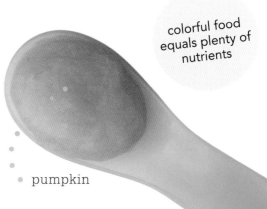

pumpkin

best first fruits . . . . . apple pear

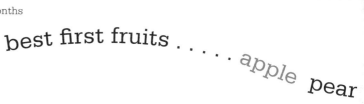

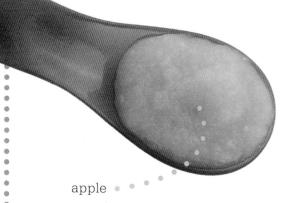

apple

Apple

Apples (see page 52) make an excellent first food for babies because they are unlikely to cause an allergic reaction and can be puréed to a very smooth consistency. They are a great source of pectin, a soluble fiber that helps your baby's body process solid food more efficiently.

Pear

Pears (see page 52) also contain pectin and have a sweet, gentle taste that babies love. They are rich in vitamin C and vitamin A, and even contain some B vitamins. Pears need to be cooked only lightly before puréeing, to preserve their nutrient content. If the purée is too runny, stir in a little baby rice to thicken it up.

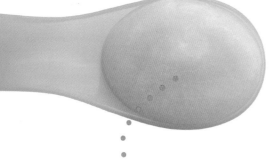

pear

ripe fruits are full of flavor and nutrients

...it's best to follow vegetable purées with fruit, as some babies may figure out that fruit is sweeter, and reject vegetables.

Banana

Sweet, ripe bananas (see page 54) are the perfect convenience food because they can be prepared without cooking, and simply mashed into a soft purée. Add a little baby milk if the purée is too thick. Bananas contain vitamin C, and the mineral potassium, which encourages your baby's muscle development. What's more, they are little packets of energy, providing three healthy natural sugars. Better still, no other fruit contains more digestible carbohydrates than banana.

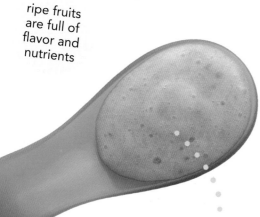

banana

banana papaya mango avocado

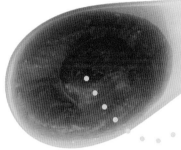

papaya

chat, smile, and sing while you feed—first foods are fun!

Papaya

Papaya (see page 54) is another fruit that can be puréed without cooking. Its brightly colored flesh is rich in vitamin C and beta-carotene, and it also contains plenty of fiber, folic acid, and vitamin E, making it a nutritious first food. Most babies love the flavor, too. Papaya contains a natural chemical called *papain*, which helps to encourage healthy digestion, and other key nutrients that encourage healthy eyesight.

Mango

Mangoes are rich in vitamins A, B, and C, and contain more calcium than almost any other fruit. They contain a little iron, too. Make sure the mango is ripe, sweet, and not stringy. Cut the mango in half on either side of the pit, peel away the skin, cut the flesh into cubes, and purée using a hand blender. Mangoes can be blended with apples, pears, or just about any other fruit to create a delicious tropical treat (see page 55).

mango

Avocado

Avocado (see page 54) is rich in healthy mono-unsaturated fats and good-quality proteins, which encourage your baby's growth and development. It also contributes nearly 20 vitamins, minerals, and beneficial plant compounds to her diet. It's a perfect, nutrient-dense first food and its smooth consistency makes it ideal for babies. There's no need for cooking, just mash it on its own, or blend with your baby's favorite fruit or vegetable purée. Slices of avocado also make good first finger foods for independent babies.

Which consistency?

Your baby's "starter" purées should be semi-liquid—almost the same consistency as yogurt. To begin with, she'll seem to suck the food off the spoon. The more liquid the purées are at the outset, the easier your baby will find them to eat.

Preparing your baby's meals

Providing your baby with healthy, nutritious meals is much easier than you may think when you first start out. Keeping in mind a few basic tips will make sure that he gets the most from the healthy food being offered.

Healthy cooking

Your baby won't be eating much to begin with, so it's important that his food is as nutritious as it can be. Choose produce that is fresh and make sure that your cooking method preserves the nutrients.

Steaming: This is a great way to preserve taste and nutrients, in particular vitamins B and C. You can place the food in a steam basket or colander over boiling water and steam until tender. Or, you can steam in the microwave.

> " *Your baby won't be eating much at the beginning of the weaning process, so it's important that his food is as nutritious as it can be.* "

Microwaves: Studies have shown that steaming food in the microwave is safe and leaves nutrients relatively intact. It is equally as good as steaming over boiling water and it's also possible to cook small quantities. Place the fruit or vegetable in a dish (or microwave steamer), cover (leaving a vent for steam), and cook on full power until tender. You can use the cooking water or your baby's usual milk to help achieve the right consistency.
Boiling: Although this does tend to rob many fruits and vegetables of their nutrient value, some foods simply don't become soft enough for puréeing using steam. Be sure to use only a small amount of water and save the cooking liquid to thin the puréed food to eating consistency.
Baking or roasting: If you are using your oven to cook a family meal, include some vegetables for your baby. Potatoes, butternut squash, sweet potatoes, and pumpkin bake to a nice consistency. Prick the vegetables with a fork and bake until tender, then scoop out the contents and purée.

Food hygiene

Keeping your kitchen clean and using different cutting boards and knives for meat and fruit/vegetables is a good way to keep food-borne illnesses at bay. Puréed food spoils more easily than other food, so must be either used immediately once prepared or placed in the refrigerator once cool, where it will stay fresh for two or three days. Purées can be frozen for future use, and will last for several months in the freezer. By the time your baby reaches weaning age, he'll be putting things into his mouth, so there is no need to sterilize spoons or containers, although they should be washed in hot, soapy water or in the dishwasher, at a temperature high enough to kill germs. It is important, however, to continue to sterilize bottles, particularly the teats. Warm milk is a perfect breeding ground for bacteria.

Puréeing your baby's food

Once your fruit and vegetables are cooked until really tender, you can purée them in a liquidizer or food processor, or with a hand blender.

Potatoes should be puréed in a mouli, or pressed through a sieve (see page 31). First foods need to be semi-liquid and similar to yogurt in consistency. Add a little of your baby's usual milk, some of the cooking liquid from the pan or steamer, or some cooled, boiled tap water to thin the purée.

Batch cooking

This involves cooking larger quantities that can be divided into portions in small containers or ice-cube trays, then frozen in batches. Get into the habit of adding extra portions of fruit and vegetables when you cook family meals. Bake an extra potato or two, or steam extra broccoli florets, for example. These can be puréed or mashed and then frozen. You can make up combinations by freezing two individual flavors, such as apple and pear, and then defrosting them and mixing them together.

Freezing and reheating

Freezing batches of baby food means you always have something fresh and nutritious on hand to feed your baby. Once you've cooked fruit and vegetables until tender, purée them and then cover. Allow to cool before freezing. Fill the ice-cube trays or containers almost to the top with the purée and store in a freezer that will freeze at 0°F (-18°C) or below within 24 hours. To thaw, take the food out of the freezer several hours before a meal and then reheat until piping hot. Allow to cool before serving. It's important to cook food thoroughly. If you use a microwave, stir carefully and watch out for "hot spots." Do not refreeze meals that have previously been frozen and defrosted. The exception to this is raw frozen food, such as frozen peas, which can be cooked and then refrozen.

Kate asks . . .

I find it easier to buy ready-made organic purées, as I don't have much time for cooking. Is there any real benefit to making baby food at home?

There is nothing wrong with relying on store-bought baby food to get you through a busy time. However, be aware that the nutritional content may be compromised because of the heat treatment necessary to make them safe throughout a long shelf life. They also tend to lack the natural sweetness and flavors of fresh foods, and giving mainly pre-prepared baby foods rather than fresh can make it more difficult for your baby to make the transistion to family meals. Although organic baby food is prepared without the use of artificial ingredients, it's worth noting that current legislation governing regular baby foods has made it almost impossible for them to contain any pesticides, so organic is unlikely to be superior in any major way.

Batch cooking, puréeing extra portions from family meals, and swapping trays of purées with friends can make it quick and easy to offer a wide range of homemade baby foods.

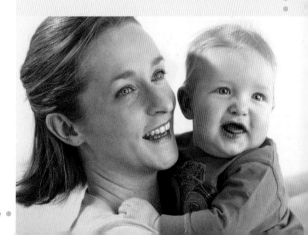

The very first spoonful

Your baby's first taste of "real" food is a momentous occasion and you'll want to choose just the right moment to make it a success. Don't be surprised, though, if things don't go according to plan. Some babies eagerly embrace those first mouthfuls, while others are a little shocked.

Where?

It's a good idea to choose a spot where you'll be regularly feeding your baby, so that she begins to associate it with mealtimes. The kitchen is probably best, as she's bound to make a considerable mess for the first few months—or even years!

In what?

If your baby is comfortable in her bouncy chair, this is perfect. Her car seat will also work well—just make sure she's sitting upright. You may already have put your highchair to use, with a cozy insert to make your young baby secure. This may make feeding easier, and as she becomes accomplished you can also use the tray for her to try food on her own. Don't forget her bib and perhaps a splat mat for under the chair or seat.

> ❝It's a good idea to avoid giving your baby her first tastes in the evening, in the event that her digestive system objects, disrupting her sleep. ❞

When?

About an hour after your baby's normal milk feed, and after she's had her nap, is a good time to start her on her first tastes in the weaning process. She won't be irritable with hunger, but she may be ready to eat. Somewhere around midday is ideal. She'll most likely be alert and happy and ready for a new experience. If she's unwell or out of sorts, leave it for another day.

Who should feed your baby?

The first spoonfuls are a bit of a momentous event, so mom and dad may want to be on hand to witness her foray into the world of food. However, anyone can successfully feed a young baby, as long as they are patient and allow her to go at her own pace. Some babies respond better to having dad offer the first spoonfuls. If your baby can smell mom's milk, she might resist her new menu in favor of the comfort of something familiar. Similarly, bottle-fed babies may be upset that they are not being offered their usual, warm treat with mom.

Which food?

Rice cereal or a plain purée of a single root vegetable mixed with a bit of your baby's usual milk is the perfect first food (see page 46). If you are breastfeeding, use a little expressed milk; if you are bottlefeeding, her formula is fine. She will be used to the sweet, creamy taste of milk and may be put off by the sight and taste of anything new. Choosing sweet vegetables, or a little baby rice with milk, makes the experience less overwhelming. It's fine to start with single-fruit purées, such as pear, but beware—your little one may enjoy the sweet taste so much, you may end up with a battle on your hands to encourage her to eat anything else.

The first feed

1 When your baby is happy and settled in her high chair, scoop up a little bit of purée on the end of her spoon and gently hold it to her lips.

2 If your baby opens her mouth, slide the spoon into it and hold it there for a few moments, so she becomes accustomed to the new taste.

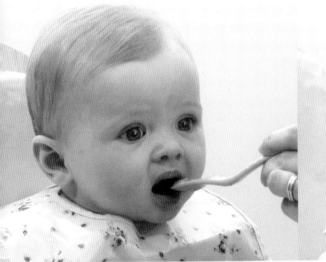

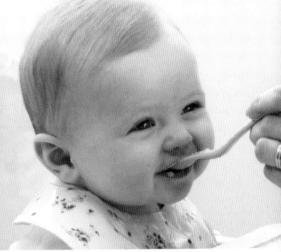

3 Carefully withdraw the spoon, using her lips and gums to remove the purée. She may suck at the spoon or even bite down on it with her gums.

4 Refill her spoon and offer a little more. Don't be surprised if most of the purée re-emerges! Simply scoop it back up and try again.

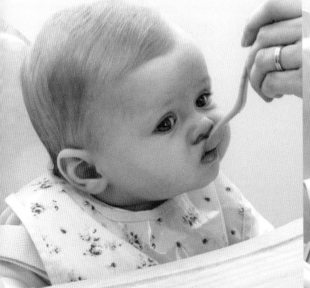

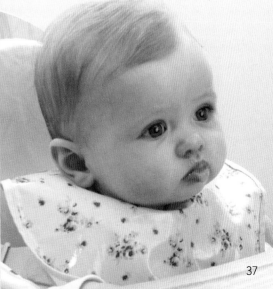

What consistency?

Adding a little of your baby's usual milk to the purée will make it seem more "familiar" as well as making sure that it is smooth and almost yogurt-like. To begin with, your baby will "suck" the food from the spoon rather than use her lips to remove it. Until she masters the art of moving the food around her mouth with her tongue, it will need to be liquid enough for her to swallow straight down.

How much?

First foods are simply tastes and her usual milk will remain her major source of nutrition. One or two tablespoons of purée is about right for the first week or so, but she may want more or less.

How often?

Once a day is perfect for the first week or two. Then experiment. If your baby is eager to move

Ready to go. Prepare your baby's first purées so that they have a smooth, yogurt-like consistency, then begin by offering just a few teaspoons per "meal," being careful not to overload the spoon.

on to two "meals," then that's fine. After a week of tastes, she may enjoy a little treat of her own when the family sits down to eat (see pages 56–57).

What temperature?

Heat your baby's purée in the microwave or in a small saucepan on the stove. Stir it carefully to make sure that it is evenly heated through, particularly if you are using the microwave, which can create "hot spots." Body temperature is just about right. Test a little on the inside of your wrist, just as you would with formula, and if you can't feel it, it's the perfect temperature. If it's too hot, set it to one side for a few minutes.

Which spoon?

Choose a narrow-headed, shallow spoon that fits easily into your baby's mouth. She may not open her mouth for those first few tastes, so your spoon will need to be small enough to slip in. A soft plastic, silicone, or rubber-tipped spoon, known as a "weaning spoon," and suitable from four months onward, will be friendlier than a cold, metal one. Choose a spoon with a shallow "bowl," so that she can easily suck off the contents. You can also give her a chunky plastic spoon to encourage her to feed herself, although she may not be able to do this properly for a while.

Which bowl?

Choose a bowl that you can grip easily, as your baby may reach out and try to grab it. A small bowl makes it easier to scoop up the contents and helps to keep them warm. If you want to get your baby involved, you can put a small portion of food in a bowl of her own and allow her to explore the contents with her hands, or with a small plastic spoon. Be prepared for mess and choose a bowl with a suction cup so that she can't pick it up.

How long should it take?

Give your baby plenty of time to get used to things in the early days. She may simply not understand what's required of her, and it may take some time for her to come to grips with the idea that there is food on the spoon. Equally, however, don't continue if she becomes bored or distressed (allow no more than 30 minutes per mealtime). Mealtimes should be fun and pleasurable, so the minute things become tense, it's time to stop.

What if she doesn't like it?

Some babies can take several sittings before they get used to the idea of having solid food. It may not be the purée your baby dislikes—it may simply be the whole process of weaning. If she expresses dislike for a particular purée, take it away and try it again in a few days. You may have to offer the same purée several times before she begins to think of it as being "familiar."

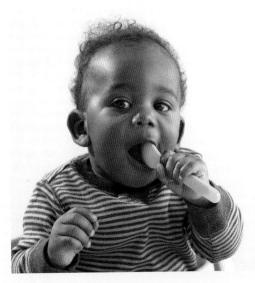

Going it alone. It's a great idea to give your baby his own spoon so he can try to feed himself—or at least chew on it.

The next few weeks

Once you've managed to get a few teaspoons of purée into your baby's mouth, you'll feel more confident about introducing new foods. But take it slowly. First foods are all about becoming familiar with new tastes and textures and the whole concept of swallowing, so your baby won't be ready for full meals for some time yet.

Introducing new foods

With most babies, you can introduce a new food every day or so, sticking with fruit, vegetables, and baby rice for the first few weeks at least. If he likes a purée, make a note (see page 21) and continue to offer it. If he doesn't seem to like something, don't give it up—simply reintroduce it a couple of days later, or blend it with a little of his usual milk and try again. Once he's tried one new food and has shown no adverse reaction, you can introduce another. If you have a history of allergies or your baby has eczema (see page 20), your doctor may suggest waiting longer between new foods.

It's perfectly acceptable to combine purées once your baby has tried a single "ingredient." So, for example, once he has mastered apple pureé you can go on to offer apple mixed with pear. Baby rice or other gluten-free cereals can be blended with any fruit or vegetable purées.

Combining breast- or bottle-feeding and solid food

Your baby will rely on his usual milk feeds for many months to come to give him nutrients and comfort. You may want to offer him "meals" halfway through a feed, or at a time when he usually has a smaller feed. His regular morning, midday, and evening feeds should continue as usual.

As he progresses toward regular meals, you can slowly reduce the number of feeds, or the length of time or amount you feed him. But play

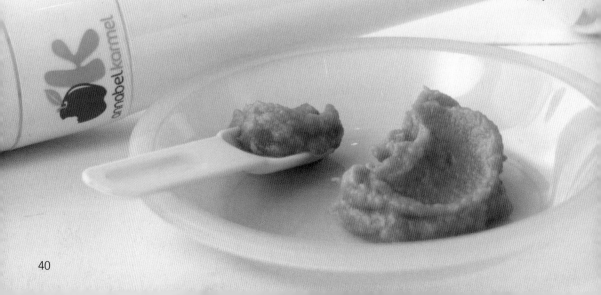

it by ear—if he's hungry, he will need to be fed. Until they are a year old, babies need at least 28oz (840ml) of milk per day. Remember that formula or breastmilk added to purées will count toward his overall milk intake. Cow's milk should not be given as a drink until after the first year, as breastmilk or formula is a better source of iron and other nutrients. However, it can be used in cooking or with cereal from six months.

Portion sizes

Don't worry too much about the amount of solid food your baby takes in. As long as he is regularly introduced to a variety of fresh, nutritious new foods, you can consider the beginning of the weaning process to be a success. You may also find that your little one is hungrier some days and eats whatever is offered, while on other days he shows little interest at all. Try to go at his pace and let his interest levels and hunger dictate how much he is fed.

As he heads toward two or three full meals a day, you will want to make sure that he is getting at least a spoonful of fruit and vegetables, a carbohydrate (such as pasta, potato, or baby rice), some protein (in the form of lentils, soy, meat, fish, or dairy products), and some healthy fats, which are also contained in dairy products, nut butters, ground seeds, and meat. The quantity doesn't matter as much as the variety.

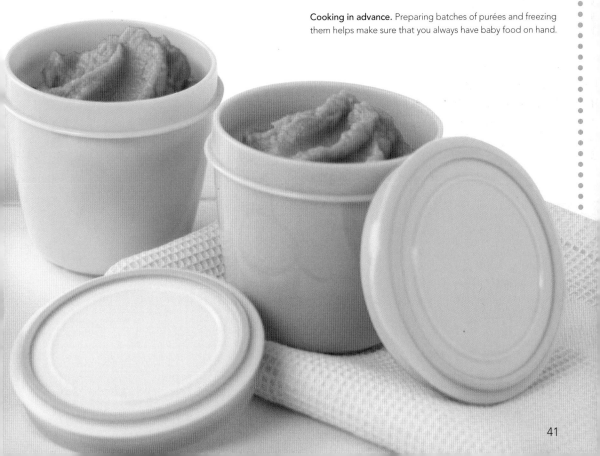

Cooking in advance. Preparing batches of purées and freezing them helps make sure that you always have baby food on hand.

Your baby's response

Even the most beautifully prepared purées can meet with resistance from your baby, and you may find that all your careful preparation goes to waste. There are, however, solutions to almost any problem that crops up. The important thing is to avoid panicking and slow down to your baby's pace.

My baby always wants more

Many parents would consider this to be a good thing, but if you are concerned that your baby is eating more than she should, or putting on excess weight, then you may want to stop her when you think she's had enough. Most babies won't want more than the equivalent of a few tablespoons of purée at the outset, although some are hungrier than others. Make sure your baby is getting enough of her usual milk—she may genuinely need more milk for her growth and development.

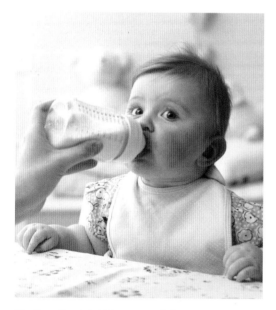

Meeting milk needs. Make sure your baby is getting enough of her usual milk (20oz/600ml) alongside her first purées.

My baby refuses to open her mouth

First of all, be sure that you aren't anxious when you are feeding her. If she senses that her clamped lips are getting a response from you, she may well continue—and even consider it a game. Try to use distraction. Get her to look up at something on the ceiling, causing her mouth to fall open. Slip in a little food and see what she does. If she resists the spoon, try either rubbing a little purée on her lips or dip a clean finger in it and allow her to suck it. You can also offer her a little bowl of purée, in which she can dip her fingers (which will eventually end up in her mouth). Try eating a little of the purée yourself—many babies are happy to mimic mom or dad!

She cries when I sit her down to eat

It might help to have another familiar person feed her. Breastfed babies in particular associate mom with the comfort of breastfeeding—they can smell her milk and may become upset when it isn't being offered. Try sitting her on your lap and holding her closely when you feed her—she may simply feel isolated on her own in a big high chair. Or, you may need to give weaning a rest for a few days—if she becomes anxious and upset, she can become increasingly difficult. Distraction sometimes helps—play games, laugh, and sing so that she associates mealtimes with fun. If all else fails, place a little purée on her tray and let her experiment herself. This way, the pressure is off.

My baby started on solids, but is now refusing them

It's not unusual for babies to regress during the weaning process. It's a big developmental leap to adjust to eating new and different foods, and to give up the comfort of milk feeds. Some babies may be slower to adjust to this change and be reluctant to continue. Try to make the process easier by offering your baby plenty of milk after her "meals." If she knows that she's still getting what she wants and that her comfort feeds have not been replaced by a hard spoon with unfamiliar contents, she'll be less likely to object. Don't give up altogether, though. Continue to offer new foods daily, but try to stay relaxed and calm if she rejects them. She'll eventually become accustomed to the new routine and look forward to mealtimes, particularly if they are fun, sociable experiences, and she is praised for her efforts.

There are solutions to almost any problem that crops up. The important thing is to avoid panicking and to slow down to your baby's pace.

My baby seems to like the purées, but not the spoon

Babies are unable to lick food from a spoon with their tongue, so make sure you are using a spoon that is soft-tipped and shallow (see page 28) so she can take some food with her lips. Give her one of her own to hold, too, so that she becomes familiar with it. Try using a piece of lightly toasted bread to scoop up some purée and let her suck that to help her get used to the idea. There is no harm in letting her try to feed herself from a small bowl or straight from her tray, using her hands.

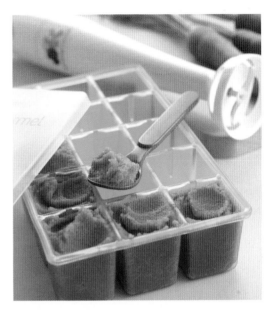

Sweet veggies first. Your baby will be used to the sweet taste of milk, so it's a good idea to start the weaning process with sweet vegetable purées.

She only likes sweet purées

Try to introduce sweet-tasting vegetables, such as sweet potato or carrots. When she seems hungrier, always begin a meal with a vegetable purée rather than fruit. Once she has mastered single purées, try blending fruits and vegetables, then gradually reduce the amount of fruit across a few days.

My baby misses the closeness of breastfeeding

Many babies find the transition from breastfeeding difficult and it's not surprising that a spoon with mysterious contents doesn't hold much allure. Try sitting your baby on your lap and holding her close. To begin, it can help to feed her a little expressed milk on a spoon, to help her adjust. From there, gradually add a little baby rice or fruit and vegetable purées.

Introducing finger foods

Finger foods are a great addition to your baby's healthy diet and you can start offering them as soon as he has had his first tastes of a range of different fruits and vegetables, and then alongside them. These foods help your baby to develop the skills he needs to feed himself and also persuade him to chew and to explore new tastes and textures at his own pace.

Moving from milk feeds to solids is quite challenging for many babies, and personally I prefer to introduce babies to different tastes and textures in the form of purées before moving on to finger foods. Purées are easy to master, easily digested, and it takes only a few weeks to make a gradual transition to eating solid food.

Good first-stage finger foods:

Depending on your baby's ability to gum and chew, the following are ideal first finger foods. Make sure he has mastered them in purée form first, so that you are sure he can manage them. The individual pieces should be large enough for your baby to pick up. Always watch him closely as he eats them.

🌟 Miniature rice cakes.

🌟 Well-steamed vegetables, such as carrot sticks and mini broccoli florets.

🌟 Pieces of well-steamed fruit, such as apple and pear (do not offer hard, raw fruit until your baby is able to bite and chew).

🌟 Hand-sized chunks of very soft, ripe fruit, such as avocado and banana.

🌟 Melt-in-the-mouth baby snacks, such as baked corn snacks.

However, once you have successfully introduced your baby to a variety of different purées, it's time to offer finger foods alongside. As he masters each new food, it can be offered in strips or chunks that he can suck, dip into purées, or simply play with.

If he gets used to having "solid" food with his purées, he'll find it easier to adapt to lumpier textures later on. Choose foods that he can easily gum to swallowing consistency and that will dissolve in his mouth. You can then graduate to foods that require a little more chewing (see page 66). Watch him closely when he's eating finger foods, as there is always a risk of choking (see page 68).

Baby-led weaning

Some parents choose to skip the purée stage altogether and opt for baby-led weaning. The idea behind this is that you miss out on the purée stage and allow your baby to feed himself right away, offering a selection of appropriate nutritious finger foods and letting him join in with family meals from the start, regardless of his ability to chew or bite. However, by giving finger foods to young babies who haven't had purées first, I am concerned that they might bite off a piece of food and choke (never leave your baby alone during or after meals). In addition, as many young babies' hand–eye coordination is not developed enough for them to be able to rely on feeding themselves, I believe they are less likely to eat the variety of foods their bodies need for healthy growth and development.

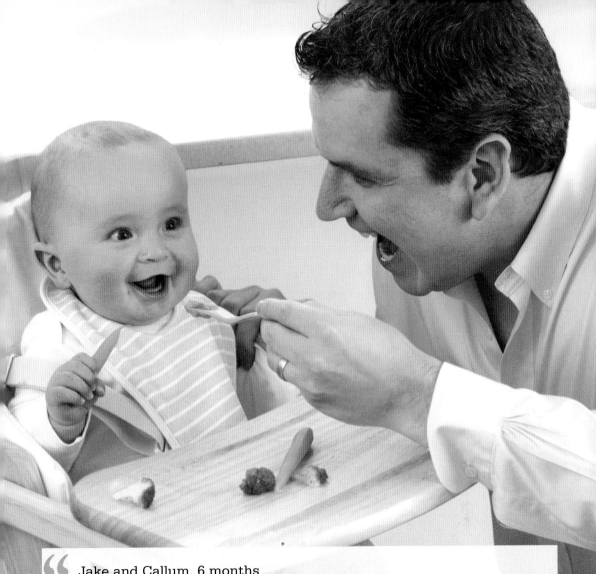

Jake and Callum, 6 months

At six months, Callum took an instant dislike to mealtimes and we were starting to worry that he'd never catch on. In fact, we could see he was sensing our anxiety and beginning to cry as soon as his highchair came into view. So, we decided to take a step back and start again. We put the highchair away and sat him in his familiar car seat. I then gave him a spoon with some fairly thick purée on the tip and let him suck that. He also had a rice cake, which he gummed up pretty well. After a few days, I managed to slip a spoonful of carrot purée into his mouth, which he didn't object to. After a week, he seemed calmer when the bowl came out and we moved him back to his highchair. We covered the tray with goodies and gave him a few different spoons to play with. He hardly noticed he was eating! I think the message is that mealtimes need to be pretty calm and anxiety-free to be successful.

First Vegetable Purée

Carrots are a perfect starter food for your baby, with plenty of nutrients and a sweet taste and smooth texture. You can prepare other root vegetables, such as sweet potato, rutabaga, and parsnip, using this method, too.

⚜ Makes 4 portions ⚜ Suitable from 17 weeks ⚜ Prep time 5 minutes ⚜ Cooking time 15–20 minutes
⚜ Suitable for freezing ⚜ Provides beta-carotene, vitamin C, folic acid, fiber

Ingredients:
2 medium carrots, peeled, chopped, or sliced
A little breast milk or formula (optional)

Method:
1 Put the carrots in a steamer set over boiling water. Cover and steam for 15–20 minutes, until the carrots are really tender.

2 Purée the carrots until smooth in a food processor or place in a bowl and use a hand blender, adding a little water from the steamer or some of your baby's usual milk to get the right consistency. First purées should be very runny so they are easy for your baby to swallow.

3 Freeze in individual portions. When needed, thaw overnight in the refrigerator or for 1–2 hours at room temperature, then microwave or reheat in a small pan until piping hot. Stir and allow to cool before serving.

Variation:
Alternatively, you can place the carrots in a saucepan, cover with boiling water, then bring back to a boil. Reduce the heat, cover, and simmer for about 15 minutes. Purée, as above, until really smooth, adding some of the cooking liquid from the saucepan or your baby's usual milk to get the right consistency for your baby.

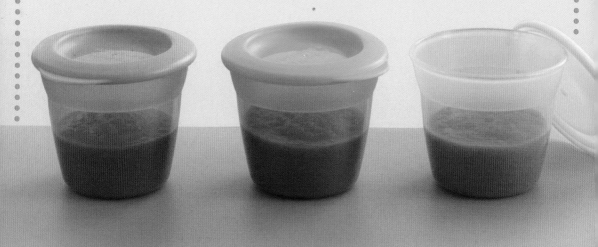

Roasted Butternut Squash or Pumpkin

Roasting root vegetables brings out their natural sugars and flavor. Both butternut squash and pumpkin make good first weaning foods, as they are easily digested and unlikely to cause an allergic reaction. Pop some in the oven when you are cooking a meal for the family, then process until smooth.

✦ Makes 6–8 portions ✦ Suitable from 17 weeks ✦ Prep time 5 minutes ✦ Cooking time 1 hour
✦ Suitable for freezing ✦ Provides beta-carotene, vitamin C, vitamin E, fiber

Ingredients:
1 small butternut squash or ½ small pumpkin
   (about 1½lb)
A little breast milk or formula (optional)

Method:
1 Preheat the oven to 350°F.

2 Halve the butternut squash. Scoop out the seeds and fibrous strings from both halves. Place the squash or pumpkin cut-side-down in a shallow oven-proof dish, and pour in some water so that it comes about ½in up the sides of the dish. Roast for about 1 hour or until the flesh is tender.

3 Remove from the oven and allow to cool. Scoop out the flesh and purée until smooth in a food processor or place in a bowl and use a hand blender. Add a little of your baby's usual milk to thin the consistency if your baby prefers.

4 Freeze in individual portions. When needed, thaw overnight in the refrigerator or for 1–2 hours at room temperature, then microwave or reheat in a small pan until piping hot. Stir and allow to cool before serving.

Variation:
You can also steam the butternut squash or pumpkin. Cut in half and scrape out the seeds and fibrous strings and discard. Peel and cut into cubes. Place in a steamer and steam for 12–15 minutes or until tender. Purée until smooth, as above.

Baked Sweet Potato

Sweet potato is a fantastic source of beta-carotene and a variety of other nutrients. Unlike ordinary potatoes, it can be easily mashed or puréed without becoming too starchy. It also freezes well.

✶ Makes 6 portions ✶ Suitable from 17 weeks ✶ Prep time 3 minutes ✶ Cooking time 1 hour
✶ Suitable for freezing ✶ Provides beta-carotene, vitamin C, vitamin E, fiber

Ingredients:
2 small sweet potatoes (about 1lb 2oz in total)
A little breast milk or formula (optional)

Method:
1 Preheat the oven to 400°F.

2 Scrub the potatoes and prick with a metal skewer or fork. Place on a baking sheet and bake for about 1 hour or until wrinkled and tender.

3 Remove from the oven, cut the potatoes in half, scoop out the flesh, and purée in a food processor or place in a bowl and use a hand blender. You can add a little of your baby's usual milk to thin the consistency if your baby prefers.

4 Freeze in individual portions. When needed, thaw overnight in the refrigerator or for 1–2 hours at room temperature, then microwave or reheat in a small pan until piping hot. Stir and allow to cool before serving.

Variation: Baked Sweet Potato and Butternut Squash
Combine baked sweet potato with baked butternut squash for a highly nutritious purée. Lay a large piece of foil on a baking sheet and spread cubes of squash and sweet potato on the foil. For babies under six months, you can brush the sweet potato and butternut squash with a little sunflower oil. For babies aged six months old and over, cut a knob of unsalted butter into pieces and dot over, then sprinkle with water. Cover with a second large piece of foil and scrunch the edges of the two foil pieces together to form a parcel. Bake for about 30 minutes or until the vegetables are tender. Cool the vegetables slightly then purée in a food processor (including any liquid). You can thin the purée with a little breast milk or formula if your baby prefers.

Trio of Root Vegetables

Any root vegetable will work beautifully in this recipe. They purée to a smooth consistency and have a mild flavor that babies love.

✳ Makes 5 portions ✳ Suitable from 17 weeks ✳ Prep time 10 minutes ✳ Cooking time 20 minutes
✳ Suitable for freezing ✳ Provides beta-carotene, vitamin C, vitamin E, fiber

Ingredients:
1 large carrot, peeled and diced
1 small sweet potato (about 9oz), peeled
 and diced
1 small parsnip, peeled and diced
A little breast milk or formula (optional)

Method:
1 Put the vegetables in a steamer set over boiling water. Cover and steam for 20 minutes until soft.

2 Purée until smooth in a food processor or place in a bowl and use a hand blender, adding a little water from the steamer or some of your baby's usual milk to get the right consistency.

3 Freeze in individual portions. Thaw overnight in the refrigerator or for 1–2 hours at room temperature; microwave or reheat in a pan until piping hot. Stir and allow to cool before serving.

Variation:
You can also boil the vegetables. Place them in a saucepan and cover with boiling water. Bring back to a boil, cover, reduce the heat, and cook for about 18–20 minutes, until tender. Purée as above.

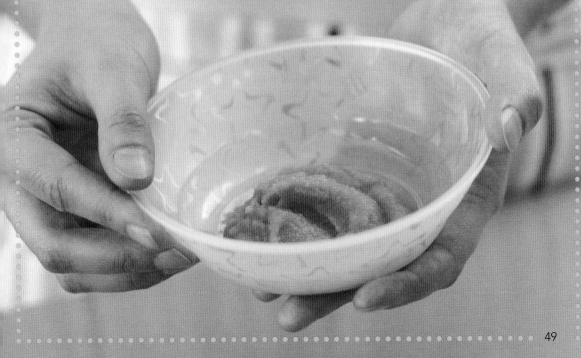

Carrot, Sweet Potato, and Apple

Combining vegetables with fruit is a great way to tempt your baby. All babies seem to love sweet tastes, and breastfed babies, who are used to the naturally sweet flavor of breast milk, will be enchanted!

✻ Makes 4 portions   ✻ Suitable from 17 weeks   ✻ Prep time 8 minutes   ✻ Cooking time 14 minutes
✻ Suitable for freezing   ✻ Provides beta-carotene, vitamin C, vitamin E, iron, fiber

Ingredients:

1 medium carrot, peeled and sliced
1 small sweet potato (about 9oz), peeled
   and diced
1 sweet dessert apple (such as Pink Lady or Gala),
   peeled, cored, and cut into small chunks
A little breast milk or formula (optional)

Method:

1 Steam the carrot and sweet potato for 8 minutes. Add the apple and steam for another 6 minutes or until all the ingredients are tender.

2 Purée in a food processor or place in a bowl and use a hand blender. Thin to the desired consistency with a little water from the bottom of the steamer or a little of your baby's usual milk.

3 Freeze in individual portions. When needed, thaw overnight in the refrigerator or for 1–2 hours at room temperature, then microwave or reheat in a small pan until piping hot. Stir and allow to cool before serving.

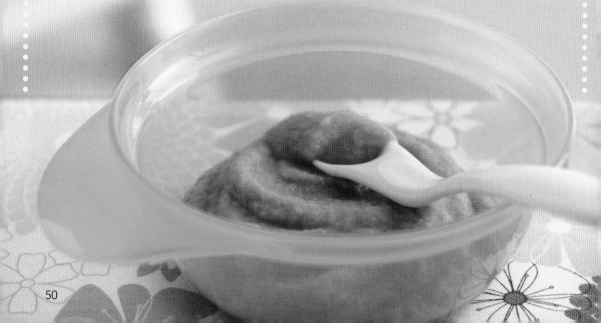

Butternut Squash and Apple

The sweet flavor of butternut squash blends beautifully with the fruitiness of apple to make this the perfect purée for even the fussiest baby.

✸ Makes 4 portions   ✸ Suitable from 17 weeks   ✸ Prep time 10 minutes   ✸ Cooking time 12 minutes
✸ Suitable for freezing   ✸ Provides beta-carotene, vitamin C, fiber

Ingredients:
½ small butternut squash, peeled and diced
   (about 3 cups)
1 sweet dessert apple (such as Pink Lady or Gala),
   peeled, cored, and cut into chunks

Method:
1 Steam the butternut squash for 6 minutes. Add the apple chunks and steam for another 6 minutes or until both are tender.

2 Purée the butternut squash and apple in a food processor or place in a bowl and use a hand blender, adding 2 tablespoons of liquid from the bottom of the steamer.

3 Freeze in individual portions. When needed, thaw overnight in the refrigerator or for 1–2 hours at room temperature, then microwave or reheat in a small pan until piping hot. Stir and allow to cool before serving.

Butternut Squash and Pear

The gentle sweetness of pears works well with any vegetable purée. Bursting with nutrients, this is an ideal first combination for your little one.

✸ Makes 4 portions   ✸ Suitable from 17 weeks   ✸ Prep time 10 minutes   ✸ Cooking time 12 minutes
✸ Suitable for freezing   ✸ Provides beta-carotene, vitamin C, fiber

Ingredients:
½ small butternut squash, peeled and diced
   (about 3 cups)
1 medium-sized ripe pear, peeled and cut
   into chunks

Method:
1 Steam the butternut squash for 8 minutes. Add the pear and steam for another 2–4 minutes, depending on how ripe the pear is.

2 Purée in a food processor or place in a bowl and use a hand blender. You probably won't need to add any liquid, but if you think the purée is too thick, you could add a tablespoon or two of the liquid from the bottom of the steamer.

3 Freeze in individual portions. Thaw overnight in the refrigerator or for 1–2 hours at room temperature; microwave or reheat in a pan until piping hot. Stir and allow to cool before serving.

Apple Purée

Apples are ideal first fruits for weaning because they are easy to digest and unlikely to cause allergies. For extra flavor, simmer the apples with a small cinnamon stick then discard it before puréeing.

✹ Makes 4 portions ✹ Suitable from 17 weeks ✹ Prep time 5 minutes ✹ Cooking time 6–8 minutes
✹ Suitable for freezing ✹ Provides vitamin C, fiber

Ingredients:
2 sweet dessert apples (such as Pink Lady, Gala, or Fuji), peeled, halved, and cored
¼ cup water

Method:
1 Dice the apple halves and place them into a heavy-bottomed saucepan with the water. Cover and cook over low heat for 6–8 minutes until really tender.

2 Purée in a food processor or place in a bowl and use a hand blender, or beat with a wooden spoon, until smooth. Freeze in individual portions and thaw as described for pear below.

Variation:
You can also steam the apples for 7–8 minutes until tender then purée—add some of the water from the bottom of the steamer or some pure apple juice to thin the purée if your baby prefers.

Pear Purée

Pears are deliciously sweet and can be easily prepared for even the smallest babies. If the purée is too runny, stir in a little baby rice to help thicken it.

✹ Makes 4 portions ✹ Suitable from 17 weeks ✹ Prep time 2 minutes ✹ Cooking time 4–6 minutes
✹ Suitable for freezing ✹ Provides vitamin C, fiber

Ingredients:
2 large or 4 small ripe pears, cored and cut into quarters

Method:
1 Put the pears in a steamer, cover, and steam for 4–6 minutes depending on ripeness. Remove, allow to cool, then peel away the skin.

2 Purée in a food processor or place in a bowl and use a hand blender, or mash with a fork, until smooth.

3 Freeze in individual portions. When needed, thaw overnight in the refrigerator or for 1–2 hours at room temperature before serving.

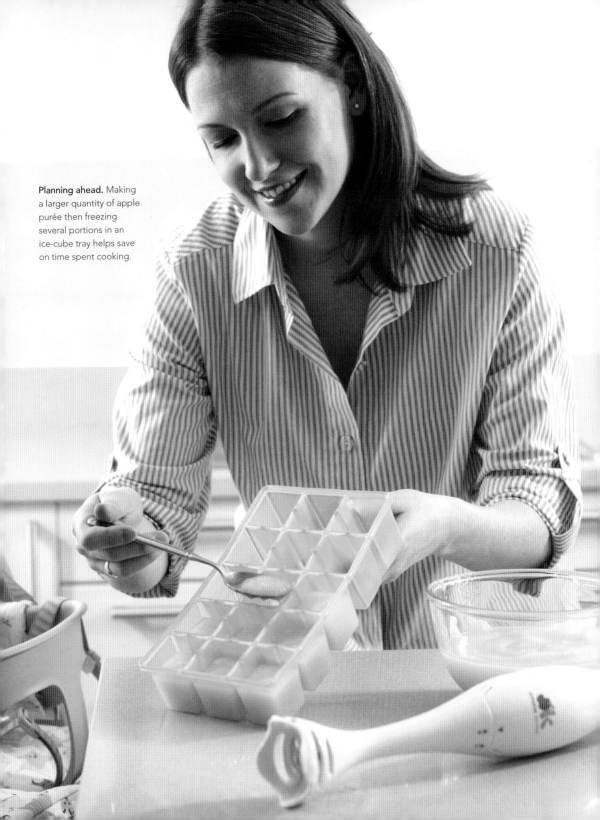

Planning ahead. Making a larger quantity of apple purée then freezing several portions in an ice-cube tray helps save on time spent cooking.

No Cook Purées

There are many purées that don't need any cooking at all. All these fruits are very nutritious and can be prepared in minutes. They each make one portion and are best eaten fresh, although you can freeze papaya if you like.

Banana

✹ Suitable from 17 weeks ✹ Provides vitamin C, B vitamins, potassium, fiber

½ small, ripe banana
A little breast milk or formula (optional)

Simply mash the banana with a fork until smooth. If the purée is too thick for your baby, you can thin it with a little of your baby's usual milk.

Avocado

✹ Suitable from 17 weeks ✹ Provides vitamin C, potassium, folic acid, EFAs, fiber

½ small, ripe avocado
A little breast milk or formula

Cut the avocado in half and remove the pit. Scoop out the flesh into a bowl and mash together with a little of your baby's usual milk.

Variation: Avocado and Banana

A popular purée combination that is very nutritious is mashed avocado and banana. Place the sliced banana and the avocado flesh into a bowl and mash together.

Papaya

✹ Suitable from 17 weeks ✹ Provides beta-carotene, vitamin C, vitamin E, folic acid, fiber

½ small, ripe papaya

Cut a small papaya in half and remove the black seeds. Scoop the flesh into a bowl and mash with a fork until smooth.

Peach and Banana

✹ Suitable from 17 weeks ✹ Provides beta-carotene, vitamin C, potassium, fiber

1 large, ripe peach
1 small, ripe banana, sliced
A little baby rice or full-fat plain yogurt

Peel the peach (see tip page 77) and then cut the flesh from the pit and mash together with the sliced banana using a fork or, if preferred, use a hand blender. If you like, you can put the peach and banana into a small saucepan and cook for a minute or two before puréeing. Serve this purée on its own or mixed with a little baby rice or yogurt.

Mango Purées

When sweet ripe mangoes are in season, they make wonderful baby food because they don't need any cooking. They are also rich in beta-carotene and vitamin C. Each recipe makes two portions and takes minutes to prepare. All are suitable for freezing apart from Mango and Banana.

Mango Purée

✹ Suitable from 17 weeks ✹ Provides beta-carotene, vitamin C, vitamin E, fiber

½ medium-sized, ripe mango

Remove the skin from the mango half and cut all the flesh off the pit to yield about 1 cup flesh. Purée in a food processor or put in a bowl and use a hand blender or mash thoroughly with a fork until smooth.

Creamy Mango

✹ Suitable from 17 weeks ✹ Provides beta-carotene, vitamin C, vitamin E, calcium, fiber

½ small, ripe mango
2 tbsp full-fat plain yogurt

Prepare the mango as for Mango Purée (see above). Place in a bowl and purée with a hand blender or mash thoroughly with a fork until smooth, then beat in the yogurt.

Mango and Banana

✹ Suitable from 17 weeks ✹ Provides beta-carotene, vitamin C, potassium, fiber

½ small, ripe mango
½ small banana

Prepare the mango as for Mango Purée (see left). Slice the banana. Purée together in a food processor or put in a bowl and use a hand blender or mash thoroughly together with a fork until smooth.

Mango and Apple

✹ Suitable from 17 weeks ✹ Provides beta-carotene, vitamin C, vitamin E, fiber

½ small, ripe mango
2 tbsp apple purée (see page 52)

Prepare the mango as for Mango Purée (see left) and place in a bowl. Purée the mango flesh together with the apple purée using a hand blender or simply mash the mango thoroughly with a fork and beat in the apple purée.

Menu planner: first tastes

My meal planners are intended as a guide only. If you prefer, you can repeat meals on two consecutive days, but it's also fine to introduce new tastes each day. Similarly, although these guides only refer to one night-time milk feed, some babies may need two.

Day	Early morning	Breakfast	Lunch	Afternoon	Bedtime
1	Breast/bottle	Breast/bottle	Carrot Purée or Baked Sweet Potato Breast/bottle	Breast/bottle	Breast/bottle
2	Breast/bottle	Breast/bottle	Roasted Butternut Squash Breast/bottle	Breast/bottle	Breast/bottle
3	Breast/bottle	Breast/bottle	Apple Purée Breast/bottle	Breast/bottle	Breast/bottle
4	Breast/bottle	Breast/bottle	Potato Purée (p31) or Rutabaga Purée (p46) Breast/bottle	Breast/bottle	Breast/bottle
5	Breast/bottle	Breast/bottle	Pear Purée with baby rice Breast/bottle	Breast/bottle	Breast/bottle
6	Breast/bottle	Breast/bottle	Carrot Purée or Baked Sweet Potato Breast/bottle	Breast/bottle	Breast/bottle
7	Breast/bottle	Breast/bottle	Roasted Butternut Squash Breast/bottle	Breast/bottle	Breast/bottle

Menu planner: when your baby is ready for more

Every baby is different, so let your baby be the guide as to when he moves on to two meals a day—hungrier babies may even like to have a fruit purée after their meal at lunchtime. You can also defrost two cubes or containers of frozen fruit purées—apple and pear, for example—and mix them together.

Day	Early morning	Breakfast	Lunch	Afternoon	Bedtime
1	Breast/bottle	Apple Purée Breast/bottle	Baked Sweet Potato or Roasted Butternut Squash Breast/bottle	Breast/bottle	Breast/bottle
2	Breast/bottle	Banana Purée Breast/bottle	Trio of Root Vegetables Breast/bottle	Breast/bottle	Breast/bottle
3	Breast/bottle	Mango Purée or Mango and Banana Purée Breast/bottle	Butternut Squash and Apple Breast/bottle	Breast/bottle	Breast/bottle
4	Breast/bottle	Apple and Pear Purée with baby cereal Breast/bottle	Carrot Purée Breast/bottle	Breast/bottle	Breast/bottle
5	Breast/bottle	Banana Purée or Papaya Purée Breast/bottle	Trio of Root Vegetables Breast/bottle	Breast/bottle	Breast/bottle
6	Breast/bottle	Apple Purée with baby cereal Breast/bottle	Carrot, Sweet Potato, and Apple Breast/bottle	Breast/bottle	Breast/bottle
7	Breast/bottle	Banana Purée or Peach and Banana Purée Breast/bottle	Butternut Squash and Apple Breast/bottle	Breast/bottle	Breast/bottle

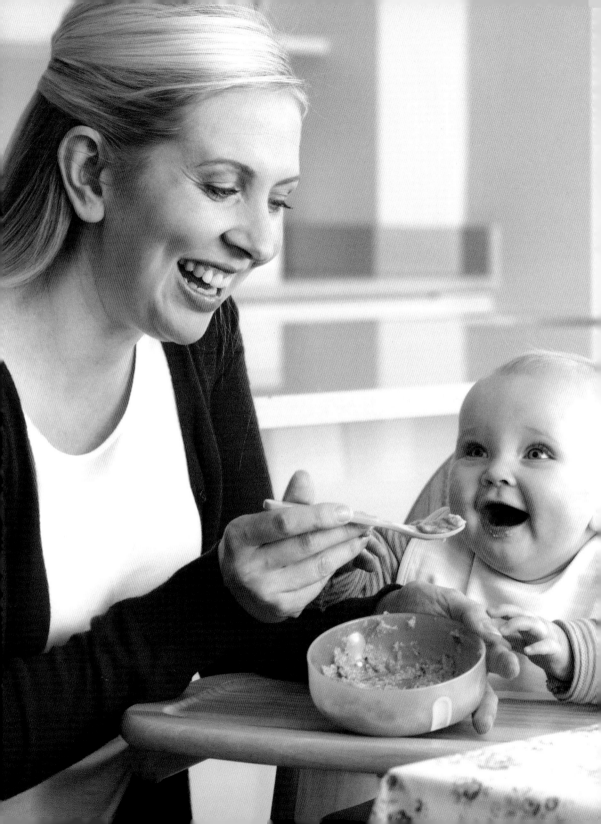

Exploring new tastes & textures

Once your baby has **learned to accept and swallow** his first tastes and has been offered plenty of **different fruits and vegetables,** it's time to move forward again. By now, your baby should be ready to **extend his repertoire** and you can add dairy products, meat, poultry, and fish, as well as an **increasing variety** of fruits and vegetables. He'll also be ready to try purées with a **little more texture,** and that means lumps!

⭐ Menu planner page 97

Getting it right from the beginning: introducing new foods

Your baby's diet can expand dramatically once she's mastered eating her first foods, but that doesn't mean introducing new foods all at once. Not only will it be easier (and gentler) for her to try new foods and lumpier consistencies slowly, but you'll also then have the opportunity to see if she experiences any negative reactions to the new foods being offered.

The second stage of weaning marks the introduction of a wide range of foods. It's not enough to continue giving just fruit and vegetable purées for more than a month or so because they are low in calories—babies grow rapidly in their first year and need nutrient-dense foods as well. Foods such as chicken and other meats are unlikely to cause an allergic reaction and are important as they provide your baby with iron. Once weaning is established, you can also start giving foods such as well-cooked eggs and fish from six or seven months—these are important foods, and if a baby is going to have a reaction to them, delaying the introduction until later will not make a difference.

"Expanding your baby's diet can be fun and rewarding, as she begins to move toward three meals per day."

Expanding your baby's diet can be rewarding and fun as she begins to move toward two or three balanced meals per day. Try poached salmon with carrots and peas or puréed chicken with butternut squash and tomato. You can sprinkle some finely grated cheese on her cauliflower purée, and her apricot purée can be blended with organic, plain yogurt. See pages 74–96 for more recipe ideas.

How much does my baby need?

This stage of weaning still involves introducing new foods, one at a time and day by day, as your little one's diet expands. If she eats just a little, that's fine. Most babies won't eat much more than a tablespoon or two of any particular purée at six months, but this can dramatically increase as her milk feeds begin to dwindle. You will be working toward giving her a diet that includes some protein, carbohydrates, fruit, vegetables, and healthy fat at every meal—and this should ideally take place by the end of about nine months. For example, cereal with milk and fruit contains protein, carbohydrates, and fruit, and chicken with potato and broccoli also contains all the food groups. This way the carbohydrates are used for energy, the protein for growth, and the vitamins for other essential body functions.

Your baby will still be getting plenty of milk in her regular feeds, but you can now think about reducing the amount you feed her at one or two feeds, and perhaps skip one altogether, to make sure she's hungry enough for her solid food.

Likes and dislikes

Even babies who have taken to solid foods can instantly develop an aversion to some foods yet demand endless quantities of others. First and foremost, try to introduce new foods at the beginning of a meal, when she's likely to be hungry. If she resists them, add a little something that is tried and tested to make the purée more familiar. A little of her usual milk stirred in will often do the trick. If she doesn't like a particular food, don't force it. Simply choose something different—but not necessarily her absolute favorite. If she gets the idea that she'll get pear purée every time she says "no" to something else, you'll struggle to get anything else into her mouth! Continue to try new foods regularly, reintroducing

those that were less successful the first few times around. Some research indicates that it can take up to 12–15 offerings for babies to accept a new food.

Consider blending together purées, gradually increasing the amount they contain of the less popular foods. You can also give your baby new foods in finger-food form (see pages 68–71), or in her own bowl, so that she can experiment at her leisure, without feeling pressured.

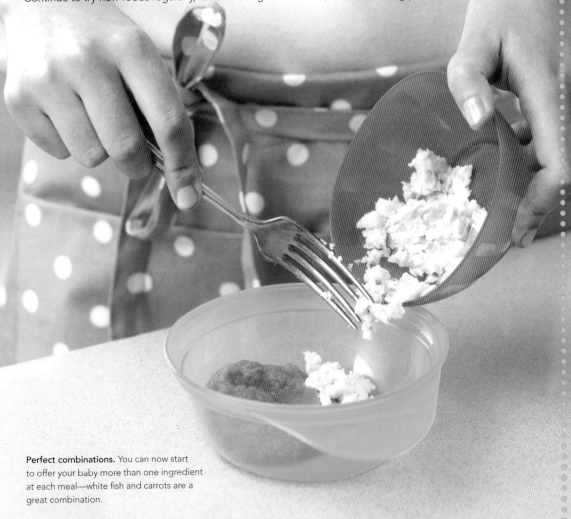

Perfect combinations. You can now start to offer your baby more than one ingredient at each meal—white fish and carrots are a great combination.

The best new foods

The second stage of weaning (around six to nine months) marks the introduction of a huge range of foods, which makes preparing your baby's meals even more enjoyable. You'll have many new options to choose from and can begin to get to work on creating truly balanced meals for your baby.

Grains and cereals

From six months, you can introduce gluten-containing grains, so oats and wheat are now on the menu. Cook oatmeal with milk and then blend with fruit purées, and offer a variety of healthy, fortified breakfast cereals. Bread is also fine, although lightly toasted bread will be easier to manage. Try stirring some well-cooked, tiny pasta shapes into your baby's purées so that she starts learning to chew. A small percentage of babies are allergic to wheat, or suffer from celiac disease (a severe sensitivity to gluten), so watch for unusual symptoms (see page 20).

Eggs

Eggs are rich in nutrients and a healthy source of protein, and can be offered from about six months. Some babies are allergic to the white, or both the yolk and the white, so introduce them carefully and cook well to reduce the risk of food poisoning. Guidelines in some countries suggest that egg whites should not be introduced until about eight months, but we now know that it can actually be beneficial to offer eggs from six months to help sensitize your baby's body to them. Eggs are a versatile food—a hard-boiled

egg can be cut up and offered as finger food, scrambled eggs make a lovely meal, and you can use eggs in cooking.

Red meat

Iron deficiency is the most common nutritional deficiency in young children. In the UK, one in five babies between six months and two years have below the desired level. Red meat provides the

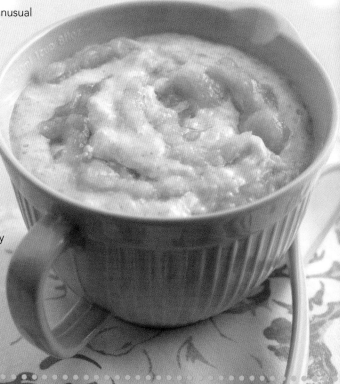

Oats are on the menu. Mix some puréed fruit into a bowl of oatmeal for a healthy, nutritious breakfast.

best source of iron as well as protein and other nutrients. Babies often reject red meat not because of its taste but because of its lumpy texture. Start with cooked lean beef or liver, which purée to a smooth consistency and combine well with fruit, such as apple or dried apricot, and root vegetables, such as sweet potato. Slowly cook lean stewing meat in a casserole with the root vegetables and fruit, and purée to a smooth consistency. You can then move on to cooked ground meat, which you can process in a blender for a few seconds to make it easier for your baby to swallow.

Chicken

Chicken is great because it is so versatile. You can combine it with root vegetables, such as carrot or sweet potato, to give it a smooth texture, or add fruit such as apple to give it a slightly sweet taste that appeals to babies. If you make a roast for the family, you could mix some of the roast chicken with cooked vegetables and some stock or a fruit purée. The brown meat of the chicken contains more iron and zinc than the breast, so it's also good to offer this to your baby. Chunks of white meat can also be offered as finger food.

Fish

The importance of fish in your baby's diet can't be overemphasized and it can be introduced at six months. We now know that the healthy fats (EFAs) contained in fish encourage growth as well as the development of your baby's brain, nervous system, and vision. Begin with mildly flavored white fish mixed with a favorite vegetable purée or a cheese sauce. You can also offer pieces of cooked fish, such as tuna, as a finger food, and oily fish, such as salmon. Aim for at least two servings a week. It's best to avoid swordfish, shark, and marlin because they may contain unhealthy levels of mercury.

Dairy products

Cow's milk, cheese, butter, and yogurt can now be included. Babies grow at a rapid rate, so you should give whole milk and dairy products. Always choose pasteurized cheeses and avoid blue cheese, Brie, Camembert, and feta until your baby reaches 12 months. Offer fresh yogurt at the end of a meal, but watch out for yogurt marketed for kids: they often contain high levels of sugar and other additives.

Fruit and vegetables

Your baby will now be able to tolerate most fruits (dried and fresh), and including a wide variety will make sure that he gets plenty of nutrients. You can continue to purée fruits, or combine fruits such as apple or dried apricot with cooked chicken or meat, or offer as a finger food. Make sure you remove all fruit pits and cut up foods such as grapes to prevent choking. Anything goes with vegetables, too, and lightly steamed vegetables make great finger foods. Both contain vitamin C, which helps your baby absorb iron, so offer them at every meal.

Legumes

Lima beans, lentils, and other dried peas and beans are a good addition to your baby's diet, offering lots of protein, iron, and fiber. Larger beans can be cooked and offered as finger food, and most beans and peas mash up well for purées—push them through a sieve if necessary to remove tough skins.

Nuts and seeds

Government advice has recently changed (see page 65). Very finely ground nuts and seeds can be offered from six months, and including them in your baby's diet may help to prevent an allergy. They are rich in EFAs and healthy proteins, too.

Foods to avoid

Although your baby will now be able to eat a wide variety of different foods, there are some that will need to wait until a little bit later. It's important to remember that your baby will not be ready for adult food just yet, and you'll need to be sure to avoid rich, fatty, spicy, salty, and sugary foods to make sure she stays healthy.

Fatty food

Babies do need plenty of fat in their diets for growth and development and to keep their energy levels high. It is, however, important to choose healthy fats (see page 15) and to avoid very fatty foods that can put pressure on the digestive system. In particular, deep-fried food is a bad idea for most babies, as are foods cooked in a lot of butter or oil.

Undercooked eggs

These can contain salmonella, which could make your baby very ill. Eggs should be well-cooked (for example, scrambled, hard-boiled, or made into an omelet) until your baby is at least 12 months old (see also page 62).

Honey

Honey is not recommended for babies under the age of one because there is a small risk of contracting botulism. Honey contains bacterial spores that produce the *Clostridium botulinum* bacteria, which make a toxin that can cause infant botulism—a rare, serious form of food poisoning. For this reason, infants under 12 months of age should never be fed honey, even if pasteurized.

Unpasteurized dairy products

Milk, cheese, and yogurt (and anything else) must be pasteurized to prevent the risk of bacterial infection. Cow's milk as a drink is not appropriate for babies under the age of 12 months, although it can be used in cooking and in other forms such as cheese, butter, and yogurt. Avoid runny cheeses, such as Brie, or those with "mold," such as blue cheese. Choose full-fat products: your baby needs the energy.

> *It's important to remember that your baby will not be ready for adult food just yet and you'll need to take care to avoid rich, fatty, spicy, salty, sugary foods.*

Artificial sweeteners, flavors, and other additives and preservatives

None of these will contribute to your baby's health and should be avoided. Fresh, whole foods should be used to create your baby's meals. Processed foods almost always contain artificial nasties, and also tend to be high in unhealthy forms of fat and sugar, so should not be offered to babies. However, if you do choose to buy jarred food for your baby, make sure you read the ingredients label carefully for non-food additives and preservatives. Ascorbic acid is okay, but make sure you avoid any others. There should be no added salt or sugar, and most definitely no transfats in the foods you buy. You'll find these listed on the label under the word "hydrogenated."

Salt

For your baby, any salt is effectively too much, so don't add it to her meal and avoid buying foods that contain it—processed meats are particularly high in salt, so avoid giving these to your baby. It might seem like an innocuous condiment, but salt can cause long-term damage to your baby's body—in particular, to her kidneys. Remember that babies aren't accustomed to salt and simply won't miss the taste, as adults might. Now is the perfect time to introduce her to the natural sweet and savory flavors of fresh foods, which she'll grow to enjoy. A tiny bit of salt used in cooking is acceptable—if you use stock cubes in your baby's purées, make sure they are well-diluted and look for low-salt or unsalted brands.

Nuts

You may be surprised to see nuts back on the menu, but guidelines have changed because there is no clear evidence that eating or not eating peanuts during pregnancy, while breastfeeding, or during early infant life influences the chances of a child developing a nut allergy. Very finely ground nuts and nut butters are a healthy addition to your baby's diet, and research indicates that early introduction may even help to prevent allergies, although more research is required. If you have a family history of allergies or eczema, watch your baby carefully. Never give whole nuts to children under five.

Sugar

It's important to introduce your baby to the natural sweetness in fresh fruits and vegetables. However, if she gets used to sugar early on, she'll not only be more likely to develop a sweet tooth and reject healthy food in favor of something sweeter, but her teeth may also be damaged. What's more, excess sugar in your baby's diet can lead to obesity in later life. Most foods contain natural sugars and provide your child with a good source of energy. Unless you need to use sugar for a particular recipe or to sweeten very tart fruit, I would recommend leaving it off the menu. It's better to choose maple syrup, agave syrup, or molasses, which offer vitamins and minerals too, or choose fruit juices or purées to sweeten.

Nitrates

Processed meats and some other foods contain nitrates, which certain experts are concerned can convert to substances that may harm your baby's health. Nitrates can also be found in some vegetables naturally, such as carrots, beets, spinach, green beans, and squash, because they are used in the soil for plant growth. Nitrates in these foods increase with storage time unless frozen, so remember to use fresh food as soon as possible and freeze extra portions as soon as they have cooled. These foods don't tend to cause problems in adults because we have higher levels of stomach acid.

Read the label

Unless your baby is from a family with a history of allergies, the introduction of most other foods should be fine. It's a good idea, however, to buy products that are clearly labeled, so you can check exactly what you are feeding your baby and to watch carefully for any reaction (see page 20).

Lumps, chunks, and learning to chew

An important part of developing speech and facial muscles is the process of learning to chew. While you might be terrified that your baby will choke if you offer food containing lumps and chunks, they do need to be added to your baby's diet—and the sooner the better!

Some babies simply don't get the idea of chewing and swallowing until they are well into their second year, whereas others are happy to chomp away on toast and chew through a variety of different textures as soon as they are offered. If your baby has a couple of teeth or a healthy set of gums, you can begin to introduce foods that are less smooth once you've established a good repertoire of purées and finger foods. Most babies are willing to give these foods a try at about seven or eight months, although you may have to wait a little longer if your baby finds them difficult to cope with.

“ Even when your baby has mastered more challenging textures and has successfully moved on to lumps and chunks, you may still need your food processor for more difficult foods, such as dried fruits, seeds, and nuts, and perhaps some tougher cuts of meat. ”

Keep an eye on your baby as he progresses and assess what he's able to manage. If he is comfortable with a variety of finger foods and can bite and chew them capably, then he is most certainly ready to have some finely chopped foods added to his normal purées.

What comes after purées?

You don't need to dispense with purées when your baby is ready to learn to chew. In fact, they form the basis of many delicious dishes and will probably remain a firm favorite for many months to come. One of the best ways to introduce texture is to stir tiny pasta shapes into your baby's favorite purées. Babies tend to prefer an overall lumpy texture rather than a smooth purée with the occasional surprise lump. You can also add mashed, ground, and finely chopped foods or tiny pasta shapes to your baby's regular purées, a little at a time—he will be familiar with the taste and maybe even intrigued by the texture!

Introducing lumps

To introduce new textures, simply mix foods with varying textures and consistency into your baby's smooth, puréed baby food. When you are cooking, put aside a little of the food before puréeing. Chop or mash it finely and stir it into the purée. Then wait to see how he does.

At first, he may spit out the lumps when he finds them in his food, but over time he'll learn to control them in his mouth, then chew, "gum," and finally swallow them. Don't rush things, though. It can take at least a week or more for your baby to get used to each new texture. If he gags or seems distressed, don't worry. Go back to his regular purées for a week or so, then try again using smaller pieces of mashed foods.

It can help to offer finger foods (see pages 68–71) alongside, which will teach your baby to put things in his mouth, then chew and swallow. It won't be such a shock then to have a lumpy purée. Don't delay, though. Babies who are introduced to lumps early on are much more likely to accept them without problems. I find that many babies will happily munch on finger foods but refuse lumpy foods on a spoon—so learning to eat lumps has more to do with habit than anything else.

Going lumpy. It's a good idea to start stirring tiny pasta shapes into your baby's purées to encourage him to chew.

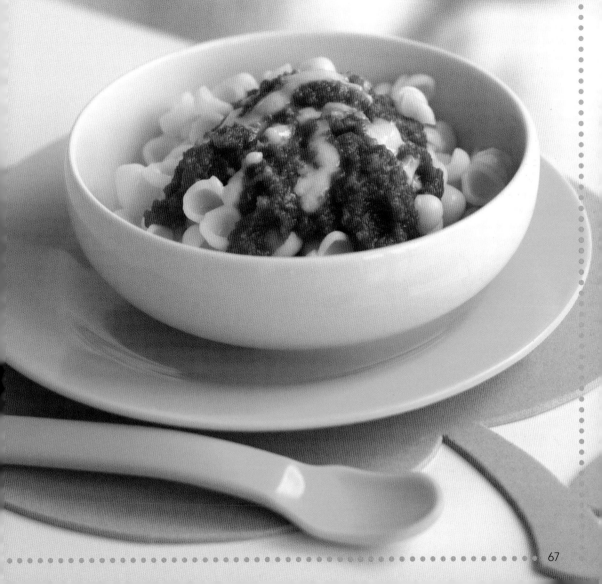

Foods for little fingers

By the time your baby reaches six or seven months, finger foods are not only a perfect way to supplement her diet and encourage independent eating, but they are also an important part of her development.

Many babies are determined to feed themselves but lack the hand–eye coordination to get food onto a spoon and into their mouths. Finger food is an ideal solution for independent babies. You may have already introduced a few melt-in-the-mouth finger foods once you felt your baby had mastered her first purées (see page 44) and now you can build on these. If not, now is a good time to start. The main thing to remember is that finger foods form a key part of your baby's diet and so should be as healthy as any element of her main meal. They are also useful to supplement the diet of fussy eaters—some babies will reject healthy vegetable purées, for example, but have no problem munching strips of roasted red pepper.

Do teeth matter?

Some babies cut their first teeth well before they are six months old, while many don't have any teeth before their first birthday. Teeth aren't actually required for chewing many foods and it's amazing what babies can get through with no teeth at all. "Gumming" can make food smooth enough for swallowing and although biting is obviously more difficult without teeth, most babies do manage with a little persistence. It is worth introducing some finger foods that will require your baby to bite off pieces and chew or gnaw. This works to stimulate her gums to keep them healthy, and helps to develop her jaw muscles in advance of speech. Picking up food and putting it into her mouth also develops fine motor skills and coordination.

Preventing choking

Many little ones bite off chunks of harder foods, but can't chew them, making choking possible. Watch for your child storing food in her cheeks.

✦ Don't give your baby finger foods if she is on her own or if she is sat in an outward-facing stroller.

✦ Avoid giving raw vegetables or chunks of hard cheese until your baby can chew them properly.

✦ Don't give fruit with pits or whole nuts.

✦ Offer large pieces of vegetables and fruit that your baby can hold. Be careful with raisins, which can stick in the throat.

✦ Peel grapes and cut them into halves; cherry tomatoes and small plums should be quartered or cut into wedges.

✦ Learn what to do if your baby does choke. First, check the inside of her mouth and remove any lodged food. Lay her face-down on your forearm, with her head lower than her chest. With your other hand, give five sharp whacks to her mid-back. If this doesn't dislodge the food, turn her on to her back and push down with two fingers on her mid-chest, making five sharp thrusts, one every three or four seconds.

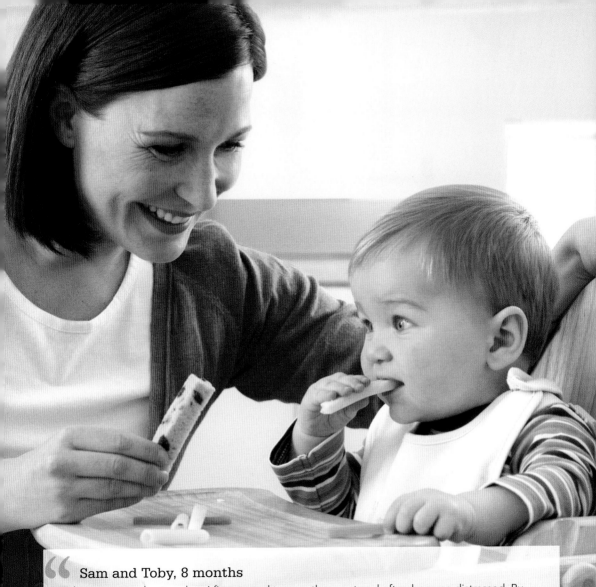

Sam and Toby, 8 months

Toby was a good eater when I first started to wean him, and he devoured most of the fresh purées I made. I felt pretty confident about including some lumpy bits and began by mashing some of the fruits and vegetables and mixing them with his usual purées. He not only refused these point blank, but spent most of the meal spitting out what I fed him. I tried all sorts of different purées, some with just one or two lumps, but he always picked them out and often became distressed. By nine months, he was still not eating lumps and I was tearing my hair out because I knew how important it was for him to chew. Eventually I solved the problem by giving him a little tray of finger foods, including some foods that I went on to purée. This did the trick. He was happy to feed himself lumpy, textured food, but he didn't want anyone messing with his purées.

best finger foods........ apples

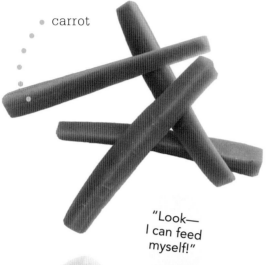

carrot

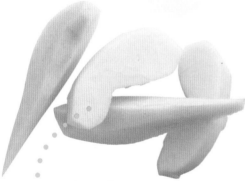

"Look—
I can feed
myself!"

apple and pear

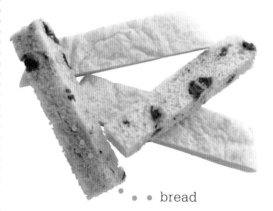

bread

Offering finger foods is an ideal way of introducing new textures, tastes, and nutrients, and is also the perfect way to encourage self-feeding. Begin by introducing foods that melt in your baby's mouth, moving on to foods that require biting when teeth emerge, or when he manages them easily.

1 Melt in the mouth

✹ Steamed-until-soft vegetables and fruit
At first, offer very lightly steamed vegetables and fruit, such as carrot sticks, mini broccoli florets, and apple and pear pieces.

✹ Very ripe fruit
Small pieces of ripe avocado and banana make perfect first finger foods.

✹ Melt-in-the-mouth baby snacks
There are many melt-in-the-mouth, salt-free baby snacks available to buy, such as baked corn or apple puffs and miniature rice cakes. These will soon become firm favorites.

2 Bite and dissolve

✹ Potatoes and sweet potatoes
Small pieces of boiled or steamed potato and sweet potato will be easy for your baby to hold. Sweet potato, especially, is packed with nutrients.

✹ Breads
You can now introduce a wide range of grains and breads. Why not offer a little pita bread, or a chunk of bagel, or sultana bread. Cut the bread into fingers or chunks, but avoid crusty breads that can break off and damage your baby's gums or cause choking. Try sandwiches made with mashed banana, cream cheese, and pure fruit spread.

pears pasta bread cheese

Eating when out and about just got a whole lot easier!

3 Bite and chew

✹ **Cucumber sticks and lightly steamed vegetables**

Cucumber sticks, as well as steamed carrot sticks, are popular with babies because they are easy to hold. Try chilling cucumber sticks in the fridge to help soothe sore gums during teething.

✹ **Cheese**

Cheese is a healthy source of fat and an excellent source of protein. Avoid very hard cheeses, which could cause your baby to choke.

✹ **Dried fruit**

Good choices are apricots, figs, apple rings, and mango. Dried fruit is a great source of iron and vitamin C. It does, however, contain lots of natural sugars. Try to look for unsulphured fruit, which does not use sulphur dioxide in the drying process. Avoid dried berries.

✹ **Mini meatballs, made from fish, chicken, or beef**

Babies love food that they can pick up and fit neatly into their mouths, and even the most lump-resistant little one will enjoy flavorful meatballs. If you are struggling to get your baby to eat meat, this may be the answer.

✹ **Fruit**

Once your baby has mastered biting and chewing, you no longer need to steam pieces of fruit. You can now introduce berries too. Berries are "superfoods," which means they contain fantastic levels of nutrients essential for optimum health.

✹ **Pasta**

You can buy pasta created from various grains, such as quinoa, wheat, and corn, and these can boost your baby's nutrient intake. If he can't eat gluten, offer rice or buckwheat pasta shapes.

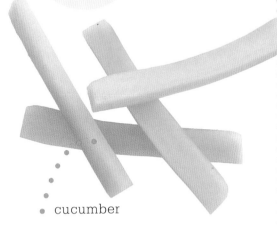

cucumber

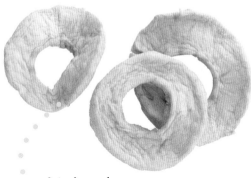

dried apple

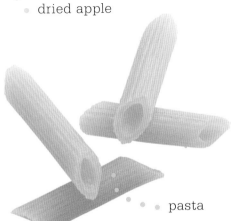

pasta

Annabel's top 10 weaning tips

Weaning isn't always a straightforward process, as babies have minds of their own—and very distinctive tastes, too! Just when you think you've got it cracked, your baby can suddenly develop eating patterns that leave you anxious and concerned. The good news is that there's a solution for everything. Keep these 10 simple tips in mind and you'll soon have your baby enjoying mealtimes and on track for a lifetime of healthy, happy eating!

1 To prevent your baby from becoming a fussy eater, try not to offer her the same purées again and again. Introduce plenty of variety, and if your little one digs in her heels, try mixing new foods with old favorites, until they become familiar.

2 Babies sleep better at night if their tummies are full and they are given foods that keep them satisfied for a longer period of time. It is therefore important for them to have a balanced meal at night that contains protein, which takes longer to digest than carbohydrates. Some protein-rich foods, such as eggs, dairy products, fish, and poultry have the added benefit of being naturally high in tryptophan, which may also help to improve your child's sleep.

3 Babies need proportionately more fat in their diet than adults, so it's important to introduce food such as meat, chicken, and cheese into your baby's diet from six months and not give only fruit and vegetable purées, which are low in calories. Don't give low-fat dairy products.

4 If your baby is putting on excessive weight, make sure you aren't pressing her to eat past the point when she has eaten as much as she wants. Babies will usually stop when they've had enough,

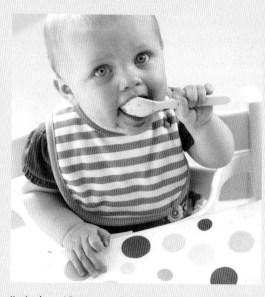

I'm in charge! Don't worry if your baby makes a mess—this is all part of learning to feed herself and also a lot of fun!

and no baby needs to clear their bowl. Consider cutting down milk feeds if your baby is getting more than 32oz (960ml) per day, and speak to your doctor or healthcare provider.

5 Allow your baby to make a mess! Not only will she enjoy eating more, but she'll be more likely to experiment with different foods, thus developing independent eating habits, when she's in charge.

6 If your baby is reluctant to try new foods, hide them in more familiar ones. For example, you can try mixing foods such as spinach or meat with sweet-tasting root vegetables. It's also good to combine savory and sweet foods such as chicken, sweet potato, and apple. Another way to introduce new foods is as finger foods, as your baby will play with them and put them in her mouth out of curiosity. Remember, it can take many attempts before she accepts a new food.

7 Go at your baby's pace. She may enjoy new foods and consistencies one day but turn her nose up the next. She may also be hungrier some days than others. Try to introduce new foods when she's happy and stick to favorites when she's grumpy. If she doesn't take quickly to new textures, lumps, or chunks, don't panic. Try some of the tips suggested in this book, and relax.

8 Make every effort to make mealtimes a positive experience for your baby. If she senses anxiety or disapproval, she'll find the experience daunting and upsetting. Praise her often, laugh, sing, and show delight at her achievements. Join her by eating a little of what she's having and she'll feel part of the family, too, and begin to associate eating with happy times.

9 Never leave your baby alone when she's eating, as she can choke on even the tiniest piece of food (see page 68). Not only that, but keeping your baby company while she's eating will teach her that eating is a sociable experience, and one to be enjoyed.

10 Plan ahead and freeze batches of foods in ice-cube trays or small containers so you don't need to cook every day.

What should my baby be drinking?

First and foremost, it's important to remember that your baby's tummy is small and if she fills up on milk, water, or fruit juice at mealtimes, she's unlikely to eat very much. It's a good idea to get your baby used to drinking from a cup, so try offering some of her normal milk feeds from a spill-proof cup (express a little, if you are breastfeeding), and offer water in one between feeds or meals as well.

It is also a good idea to offer water or milk at the end of a meal. Very dilute fruit juice can be given if your baby does not drink enough water or if you don't have a fruit or vegetable high in vitamin C on the menu to increase iron absorption. Don't offer full-strength fruit juice, as this will not only fill her up but will also encourage a sweet tooth. Furthermore, fruit juice should be limited to mealtimes and to about 4oz (120ml) per day.

Alongside this, your baby will still need her usual milk feeds, which provide her with the nutrients she needs to grow and develop.

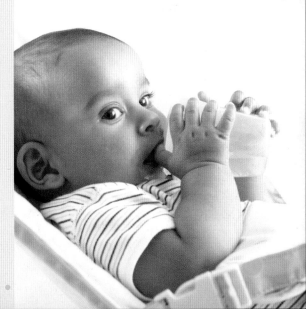

Sweet Potato with Broccoli and Peas

A good way to introduce green vegetables, such as broccoli, is to mix them with sweet-tasting root vegetables.

✹ Makes 4 portions ✹ Suitable from 6 months ✹ Prep time 5 minutes ✹ Cooking time 14 minutes
✹ Suitable for freezing ✹ Provides beta-carotene, B vitamins, vitamin C, folic acid, fiber

Ingredients:
1 sweet potato (about 1lb), peeled and diced
2 broccoli florets (about 2oz), halved
3 tbsp frozen peas

Method:
1 Steam the sweet potato for 6 minutes. Add the broccoli and steam for another 4 minutes. Add the peas and continue for 4 minutes more.

2 Purée in a food processor or put in a bowl and use a hand blender, adding enough water from the steamer to make a smooth consistency.

3 Freeze in individual portions. When needed, thaw overnight in the refrigerator or for 1–2 hours at room temperature, then microwave or reheat in a small pan until piping hot. Stir and allow to cool before serving.

Pumpkin and Pea Purée

Not only is this deliciously smooth purée highly nutritious, but it also has a sweet, mild flavor that your baby will love.

✹ Makes 4 portions ✹ Suitable from 6 months ✹ Prep time 10 minutes ✹ Cooking time 17 minutes
✹ Suitable for freezing ✹ Provides beta-carotene, vitamin C, iron, zinc, folic acid, fiber

Ingredients:
1 tbsp unsalted butter
1in piece leek, thinly sliced
2¼ cups peeled and diced pumpkin
½ cup unsalted vegetable stock or water
3 tbsp frozen peas

Method:
1 Melt the butter in a saucepan and sauté the leek gently, stirring, for 3 minutes or until softened. Add the pumpkin and cook gently for 1 minute. Pour over the stock or water, bring back to a boil, reduce the heat, cover, and simmer for 10 minutes. Add the peas and cook for 3 minutes. Purée in a food processor or use a hand blender.

2 Freeze in individual portions. Thaw overnight in the refrigerator or for 1–2 hours at room temperature; microwave or reheat in a pan until piping hot. Stir and allow to cool before serving.

Potato, Carrot, and Corn

Root vegetables, such as potatoes and carrots, are firm favorites with babies, and the fruitiness of corn makes this purée irresistible.

★ Makes 4 portions   ★ Suitable from 6 months   ★ Prep time 10 minutes   ★ Cooking time 18 minutes
★ Suitable for freezing   ★ Provides beta-carotene, vitamin C, potassium, B vitamins, fiber

Ingredients:

1 tbsp olive oil
½ small onion, peeled and chopped
1 medium carrot, peeled and sliced
1 large potato, peeled and diced
⅔ cup unsalted vegetable stock or water
3 tbsp frozen or canned naturally sweet corn,
   packed in water, drained

Method:

1 Heat the oil and sauté the onion and carrot gently for 5 minutes, stirring.

2 Add the potato, pour over the stock or water, and bring to a boil. Cover, reduce the heat, and simmer for 10 minutes or until tender. Add the corn and cook for another 3 minutes.

3 Purée in a baby food grinder or mouli or place in a bowl and use a hand blender.

4 Freeze in individual portions. Thaw overnight in the refrigerator or for 1–2 hours at room temperature; microwave or reheat in a pan until piping hot. Stir and allow to cool before serving.

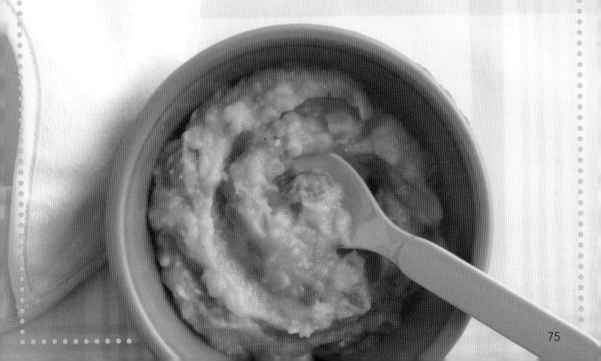

Cheesy Leek, Sweet Potato, and Cauliflower

Adding cheese to your baby's purées is an excellent way to ensure a concentrated source of calories that will help fuel her rapid growth in the first year. This tasty purée is bursting with fall-time flavors.

★ Makes 4 portions   ★ Suitable from 6 months   ★ Prep time 5 minutes   ★ Cooking time 13 minutes
★ Suitable for freezing   ★ Provides beta-carotene, vitamin C, calcium, folic acid, EFAs, fiber

Ingredients:

2 tsp unsalted butter
2in piece of leek, sliced
½ small sweet potato, peeled and diced
    (about 1⅓ cups)
1 cup boiling water
2 good-sized cauliflower florets, cut into
    4 small pieces
¼ cup shredded Monterey Jack or Cheddar cheese

Method:

1 Heat the butter in a pan and add the leek. Sauté gently until softened, about 3 minutes.

2 Add the sweet potato, pour the boiling water over the top, bring back to a boil, and cook for 5 minutes. Add the cauliflower, reduce the heat to medium, cover, and continue to cook for another 5 minutes.

3 Purée the contents of the pan in a food processor together with the shredded cheese.

4 Freeze in individual portions. Thaw overnight in the refrigerator or for 1–2 hours at room temperature; microwave or reheat in a pan until piping hot. Stir and allow to cool before serving.

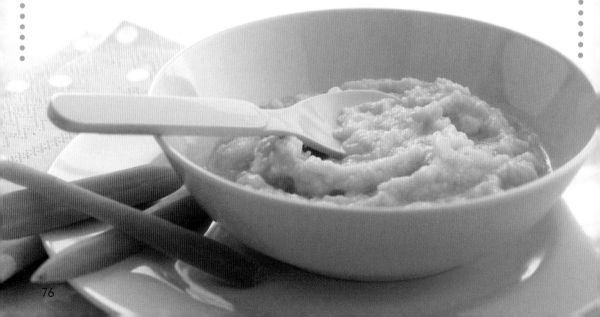

Lentil Purée with Sweet Potato

You may be surprised to hear that lentil purées are some of my most popular baby recipes. Lentils are an excellent source of protein and iron, and they also contain fiber. What's more, babies love them!

✳ Makes 3 portions ✳ Suitable from 6 months ✳ Prep time 10 minutes ✳ Cooking time 30 minutes
✳ Suitable for freezing ✳ Provides protein, beta-carotene, vitamin C, B vitamins, iron, fiber

Ingredients:

1 tbsp sunflower oil
1 small onion, peeled and chopped
¼ red bell pepper, cored, seeded, and chopped
1 medium tomato, skinned (see tip, right), seeded, and coarsely chopped
2 tbsp red lentils
½ small sweet potato, peeled and diced (about 1⅓ cups)
Scant 1 cup unsalted vegetable stock or water

Method:

1 Heat the oil in a pan and sauté the onion and red bell pepper gently, stirring, for 4 minutes until softened. Add the tomato and sauté, stirring, for 1 minute.

2 Rinse the lentils, add them to the pan along with the sweet potato, and pour over the vegetable stock or water. Bring to a boil, reduce the heat, cover, and simmer for 20–25 minutes or until the lentils are quite mushy. Top off with a little more water if necessary, but there should be only a little liquid left in the pan at the end.

3 Purée until smooth in an food processor or place in a bowl and use a hand blender.

4 Freeze in individual portions. When needed, thaw overnight in the refrigerator or for 1–2 hours at room temperature, then microwave or reheat in a small pan until piping hot. Stir and allow to cool before serving.

Tip:

The best way to peel tomatoes as well as other thick-skinned fruits, such as peaches, nectarines, and plums, is to first cut a shallow cross on the bottom of the piece of fruit using a small, sharp knife. Place the fruit in a bowl, cover with boiling water, then leave for 30 seconds to a minute. Drain and then rinse under a cold tap. When the fruit is cool enough to handle, find the cross you made in the base. Grasp a corner of loose skin between your thumb and the knife and gently pull off the skin. Repeat until all the skin has been removed.

Tomato and Butternut Squash Pasta

Rich, sweet, and full of antioxidants and other nutrients, this creamy pasta dish will appeal to babies and children of all ages. The sauce can be frozen separately in individual portions, then thawed, reheated, and served with freshly cooked pasta, potatoes, or rice.

✸ Makes 5 portions ✸ Suitable from 6 months ✸ Prep time 10 minutes ✸ Cooking time 40 minutes
✸ Suitable for freezing ✸ Provides carbohydrates, protein, beta-carotene, vitamin C, B vitamins, calcium, fiber

Ingredients:

2 tsp olive oil
½ small red onion, peeled and finely chopped
1 tsp fresh chopped thyme, or ¼ tsp dried thyme
Generous 1 cup peeled and diced butternut
    squash
1 garlic clove, peeled and crushed
14oz can chopped tomatoes
¼ cup water
½ tsp sun-dried tomato paste
¼ cup shredded Monterey Jack Cheddar cheese
1 tbsp heavy cream

To serve:
Generous ½ cup conchigliette (baby pasta shells)

Method:

1 Heat the oil in a saucepan. Add the onion, thyme, and butternut squash. Sauté, stirring, over low heat for 5 minutes. Add the garlic and cook for another minute.

2 Add the remaining ingredients except the cheese and cream. Bring to a boil, reduce the heat, and simmer gently for 30 minutes or until soft and pulpy, stirring occasionally.

3 Add the cheese and purée the mixture until smooth in a food processor or place in a bowl and use a hand blender. Mix in the cream.

4 Meanwhile, cook the pasta in boiling water according to the package directions, then drain. Stir in the tomato and butternut squash sauce before serving.

5 Freeze in individual portions. When needed, thaw overnight in the refrigerator or for 1–2 hours at room temperature, then microwave or reheat in a small pan until piping hot. Stir and allow to cool before serving.

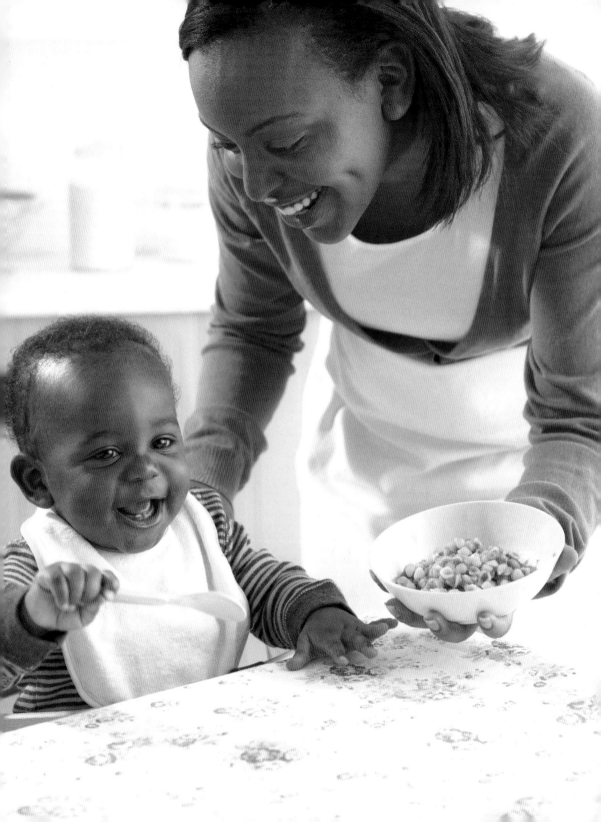

Salmon and Corn Chowder

This nourishing chowder makes a perfect meal for a hungry baby. In fact, the whole family will enjoy the rich, delicious flavors.

✸ Makes 5 portions ✸ Suitable from 6 months ✸ Prep time 10 minutes ✸ Cooking time 20 minutes ✸ Suitable for freezing ✸ Provides protein, carbohydrates, beta-carotene, vitamin D, calcium, EFAs, iron, fiber

Ingredients:
1 tbsp olive oil
1 small onion, peeled and chopped
2 medium carrots, peeled and diced
½ celery rib, strings removed (see tip, below) and chopped
1 medium potato, peeled and diced
1 small garlic clove, peeled and crushed
Scant ½ cup unsalted vegetable stock or water
Scant ½ cup milk
4oz boneless salmon fillet, skinned and cut into small cubes
3½oz canned naturally sweet corn packed in water, drained

Method:
1 Heat the oil in a saucepan. Stir in the onion, carrot, celery, and potato. Reduce the heat as low as possible, cover, and cook very gently for 10 minutes, stirring occasionally. Add the garlic and stir for 30 seconds.

2 Add the stock or water, bring to a boil, cover, and cook for 8 minutes until tender. Add the milk, salmon, and corn, and bring back to a boil. Reduce the heat again and cook gently for another 2 minutes.

3 Purée until smooth in a food processor or place in a bowl and use a hand blender. For older babies, mash with a fork.

4 Freeze in individual portions. When needed, thaw overnight in the refrigerator or for 1–2 hours at room temperature, then microwave or reheat in a small pan until piping hot. Stir and allow to cool before serving.

Tip:
The easy way to remove strings from celery is to peel the ribs with a potato peeler. This prevents unpleasant strands from appearing in the finished dish.

Poached Salmon with Carrots and Peas

It's hard to find a jar of baby purée that contains oily fish such as salmon, yet the essential fatty acids in oily fish are particularly important for the development of your baby's brain, nervous system, and vision, and ideally should be included in his diet twice a week. Did you know that fats such as these are also one of the principal sources of calories in breast milk?

✷ Makes 3 portions ✷ Suitable from 6 months ✷ Prep time 8 minutes ✷ Cooking time 11 minutes
✷ Suitable for freezing ✷ Provides carbohydrates, protein, beta-carotene, vitamin D, calcium, EFAs, fiber

Ingredients:
⅔ cup unsalted vegetable stock or water
1 small potato, peeled and diced
1 medium carrot, peeled and diced
3½oz boneless salmon fillet, skinned and cut
  into small cubes
2 tbsp frozen peas
⅓ cup shredded Monterey Jack or Cheddar
  cheese

Method:
1 Put the stock or water in a saucepan with the potato and carrot. Bring to a boil, then cook over medium heat for 7–8 minutes or until the potato and carrot are just tender.

2 Add the salmon and peas. Cover again and simmer for 3 minutes until the fish flakes easily and the vegetables are tender. Remove from the heat and stir in the shredded cheese.

3 Purée until smooth in a food processor or place in a bowl and use a hand blender. For older babies, mash with a fork.

4 Freeze in individual portions. When needed, thaw overnight in the refrigerator or for 1–2 hours at room temperature, then microwave or reheat in a small pan until piping hot. Stir and allow to cool before serving.

Annabel's Tasty Salmon

It's never too early to establish oily fish on the menu, and this salmon purée provides lots of EFAs to encourage healthy growth and development.

✹ Makes 2 portions ✹ Suitable from 6 months ✹ Prep time 5 minutes ✹ Cooking time 15 minutes
✹ Suitable for freezing ✹ Provides protein, beta-carotene, vitamin D, calcium, EFAs, iron, fiber

Ingredients:

1 large carrot, peeled and diced
3½oz boneless salmon fillet, skinned
1 tbsp milk
1 tbsp unsalted butter
2 good-sized ripe tomatoes, skinned (see tip,
    page 77), seeded, and coarsely chopped
¼ cup shredded Monterey Jack or Cheddar cheese

Method:

1 Steam the carrot for 15 minutes or until tender.

2 Place the salmon in a small microwaveable dish, add the milk, cover with plastic wrap rolled back at one edge, and microwave for 1½ minutes until the fish is just opaque. Leave to stand—it will finish cooking while you prepare the rest of the dish.

3 Melt the butter in a saucepan and sauté the tomatoes, stirring until pulpy (about 3 minutes). Remove from the heat and stir in the shredded cheese until melted.

4 Flake the fish and mix this together with the tomato and cheese sauce and the diced carrot. If your baby isn't ready for lumps yet, process the mixture in the food processor.

5 Freeze in individual portions. Thaw overnight in the refrigerator or for 1–2 hours at room temperature; microwave or reheat in a pan until piping hot. Stir and allow to cool before serving.

Cod with Butternut Squash and Cheese Sauce

Cheese sauce is a good complement to butternut squash and, depending on your baby's tastes, you can use any cheese you like, provided it is pasteurized. Sole or haddock make a great alternative to cod, and are equally nutritious and baby friendly. Add a little less milk for older babies.

✹ Makes 4 portions ✹ Suitable from 6 months ✹ Prep time 10 minutes ✹ Cooking time 11 minutes
✹ Suitable for freezing ✹ Provides protein, beta-carotene, vitamin C, calcium, iron, EFAs

Ingredients:

1 tbsp unsalted butter
½ small onion, peeled and finely chopped
3oz peeled and diced butternut squash
2 tbsp all-purpose flour
¼ cup milk
¼ cup unsalted vegetable stock or water
3½oz boneless cod fillet or other white fish, skinned and cut into small cubes
¼ cup freshly shredded Parmesan cheese

Method:

1 Melt the butter in a saucepan and stir in the onion and butternut squash. Reduce the heat as low as possible, cover, and cook very gently for 5 minutes until soft, stirring occasionally.

2 Stir in the flour and cook for 1 minute. Remove from the heat, gradually add the milk and stock or water, return to the heat, bring to a boil, and simmer for 2 minutes, stirring.

3 Add the cubes of fish and cook for about 2½ minutes until tender and cooked through.

4 Add the cheese and purée the mixture until smooth in a food processor or place in a bowl and use a hand blender. For older babies, mash with a fork.

5 Freeze in individual portions. Thaw overnight in the refrigerator or for 1–2 hours at room temperature; microwave or reheat in a pan until piping hot. Stir and allow to cool before serving.

Spinach and Cod Purée

This flavorful fish purée is packed with protein, iron, vitamin C, and antioxidants, making it the perfect way to make sure your baby gets the nutrients she needs. Skip the puréeing stage and top with mashed potatoes for a delicious family fish pie.

✹ Makes 3 portions   ✹ Suitable from 6 months   ✹ Prep time 8 minutes   ✹ Cooking time 16 minutes
✹ Suitable for freezing   ✹ Provides protein, carbohydrates, beta-carotene, vitamin C, vitamin D, iron, calcium

Ingredients:
1 tbsp unsalted butter
2in piece of leek, finely sliced
1 medium potato, peeled and diced
Scant ½ cup unsalted vegetable stock or water
¼ cup milk
2 handfuls baby spinach leaves, coarsely chopped
3½oz boneless cod fillet or other white fish,
   skinned and cut into small cubes
2 tbsp freshly shredded Parmesan cheese

Method:
1 Heat the butter in a saucepan. Add the leek and sauté gently, stirring, for 3 minutes. Add the potato and sauté, stirring, for 2 minutes.

2 Add the stock or water and milk. Bring to a boil, reduce the heat, cover, and simmer for 8 minutes, until the vegetables are tender.

3 Add the spinach and cod and stir over the heat for 3 minutes or until the spinach has wilted and the cod is cooked. Stir in the cheese and purée until smooth in a food processor or place in a bowl and use a hand blender. For older babies, mash with a fork.

4 Freeze in individual portions. When needed, thaw overnight in the refrigerator or for 1–2 hours at room temperature, then microwave or reheat in a small pan until piping hot. Stir and allow to cool before serving.

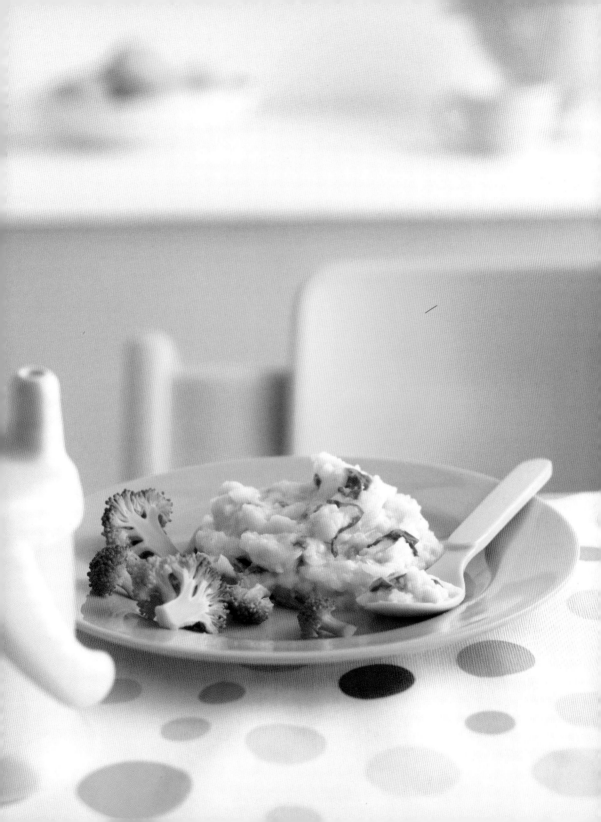

Chicken and Parsnip Purée

Chicken is often a firm favorite with babies, and it blends well with the soft consistency and mild fruitiness of puréed parsnip. If you wish, you can replace the chicken breast with boneless chicken thighs, which are higher in zinc and iron. This easy purée also freezes well.

★ Makes 4 portions ★ Suitable from 6 months ★ Prep time 8 minutes ★ Cooking time 15 minutes
★ Suitable for freezing ★ Provides protein, beta-carotene, vitamin C, zinc, iron, folic acid, fiber

Ingredients:

2 tsp sunflower oil
2in piece of leek, sliced
1 small chicken breast, cut into small cubes
1 small parsnip, peeled and diced
¾ cup peeled and diced butternut squash
½ small apple, shredded
1 cup unsalted fresh chicken stock or water
Good pinch fresh chopped thyme, or small
    pinch dried thyme

Method:

1 Heat the oil in a saucepan. Add the leek and sauté gently, stirring, for 3 minutes. Add the chicken and sauté for 2 minutes.

2 Add the remaining ingredients, bring to a boil, cover, reduce the heat, and simmer gently for 8–10 minutes until all of the vegetables are soft and the chicken is cooked through.

3 Purée until smooth in a food processor or place in a bowl and use a hand blender. For older babies, chop in a food processor or by hand to the desired consistency.

4 Freeze in individual portions. When needed, thaw overnight in the refrigerator or for 1–2 hours at room temperature, then microwave or reheat in a small pan until piping hot. Stir and allow to cool before serving.

Mild Chicken and Apricot Curry

You will be amazed at some of the flavors that will appeal to your baby, so be sure to introduce mild spices to add variety to her diet.

✴ Makes 3–4 portions ✴ Suitable from 6 months ✴ Prep time 10 minutes ✴ Cooking time 17 minutes
✴ Suitable for freezing ✴ Provides protein, beta-carotene, vitamin C, iron, EFAs, fiber

Ingredients:

1 tbsp sunflower oil
1 small onion, peeled and chopped
¼ tsp fresh ginger, shredded (optional)
1½ tsp mild curry paste
Scant ½ cup unsalted fresh chicken stock
　　or water
Scant ½ cup coconut milk
4 dried apricots, coarsely chopped
¼ small butternut squash, peeled and finely diced
　　(about 1⅓ cups)
1 small chicken breast, cut into small cubes

Method:

1 Heat the oil in a saucepan. Add the onion and ginger, if using, and sauté gently, stirring for 5 minutes. Add the curry paste and sauté, stirring for 30 seconds.

2 Add the remaining ingredients, bring to a boil, reduce the heat, cover, and simmer for about 12 minutes until the squash is tender and the chicken is cooked through.

3 Purée until smooth in a food processor or place in a bowl and use a hand blender. For older babies, chop in a food processor or by hand to the desired consistency.

4 Freeze in individual portions. Thaw overnight in the refrigerator or for 1–2 hours at room temperature; microwave or reheat in a pan until piping hot. Stir and allow to cool before serving.

Tip:

You can freeze the remainder of the can of coconut milk for use on another day.

Chicken with Sweet Potato, Peas, and Basil

This is a delicious combination purée, and the addition of garlic and fresh herbs works to bring out the natural flavors. It's also full of nutrients, such as beta-carotene, fiber, protein, and antioxidants, to encourage healthy growth and development.

✷ Makes 5 portions   ✷ Suitable from 6 months   ✷ Prep time 6 minutes   ✷ Cooking time 20 minutes
✷ Suitable for freezing   ✷ Provides protein, carbohydrates, beta-carotene, vitamin C, iron, zinc, folic acid, fiber

Ingredients:

1½ tbsp olive oil
1 small onion, peeled and chopped
½ small red bell pepper, seeded and diced
1 garlic clove, peeled and crushed
1 small chicken breast, cut into small cubes
2 tbsp pure apple juice
¾ cup unsalted fresh chicken stock or water
1 medium zucchini, diced
½ small sweet potato, peeled and diced (about
    1⅓ cups)
¼ cup frozen peas
6 fresh basil leaves, chopped

Method:

1 Heat the olive oil in a saucepan and sauté the onion and red bell pepper, stirring, for 4 minutes until softened. Add the garlic and sauté for 1 minute.

2 Stir in the chicken and continue to cook for 2–3 minutes, stirring. Pour over the apple juice and stock or water and stir in the zucchini and sweet potato. Bring to a boil, cover, reduce the heat, and simmer gently for 8 minutes. Stir in the peas and continue to cook for 3 minutes until everything is tender and cooked through. Stir in the basil.

3 Purée in a food processor or place in a bowl and use a hand blender. For older babies, chop in a food processor or by hand to the desired consistency.

4 Freeze in individual portions. When required, thaw overnight in the refrigerator or for 1–2 hours at room temperature, then microwave or reheat in a small pan until piping hot. Stir and allow to cool before serving.

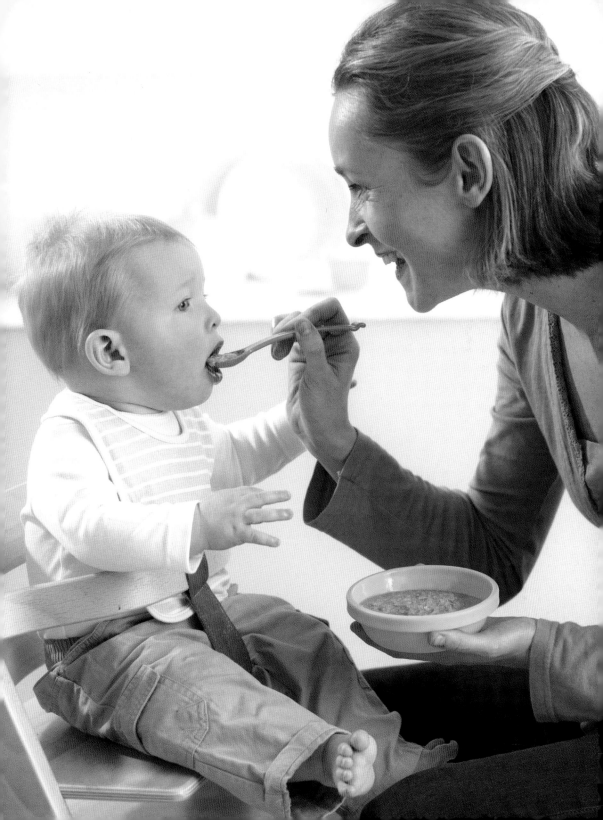

Beginner's Beef Ragout

Beef is a good source of easily absorbed iron, which your baby needs for healthy growth, development, and optimum energy levels.

✻ Makes 5 portions ✻ Suitable from 6 months ✻ Prep time 10 minutes ✻ Cooking time 1 hour 10 minutes
✻ Suitable for freezing ✻ Provides carbohydrates, protein, beta-carotene, vitamin C, zinc, iron, fiber

Ingredients:

1 tbsp olive oil
1 small onion, peeled and chopped
1 garlic clove, peeled and crushed
4oz lean stewing steak, trimmed of fat
   and cut into small cubes
1 large carrot, peeled and diced

1 large potato, peeled and diced
3 dried apricots, chopped
⅔ cup puréed tomatoes
About 1 cup unsalted chicken or vegetable
   stock or water

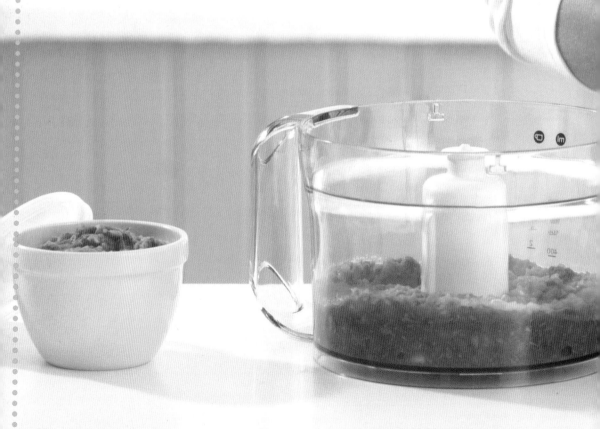

Method:

1 Heat the oil in a small flameproof Dutch oven or heavy-bottomed saucepan and sauté the onion gently for 3 minutes, stirring. Add the garlic and sauté for 30 seconds. Add the stewing steak and sauté, stirring, until browned all over.

2 Add the carrot, potato, and dried apricots, and pour over the tomatoes and stock or water. Bring to a boil, stir well, reduce the heat as low as possible, cover, and simmer gently for about 1 hour, until the meat is tender, adding a little more stock or water if necessary and stirring occasionally.

3 Cool slightly, then purée in a food processor, or place in a bowl and use a hand blender. For older babies, chop in a food processor or by hand to the desired consistency.

4 Freeze in individual portions. When needed, thaw overnight in the refrigerator or for 1–2 hours at room temperature, then microwave or reheat in a small pan until piping hot. Stir and allow to cool before serving.

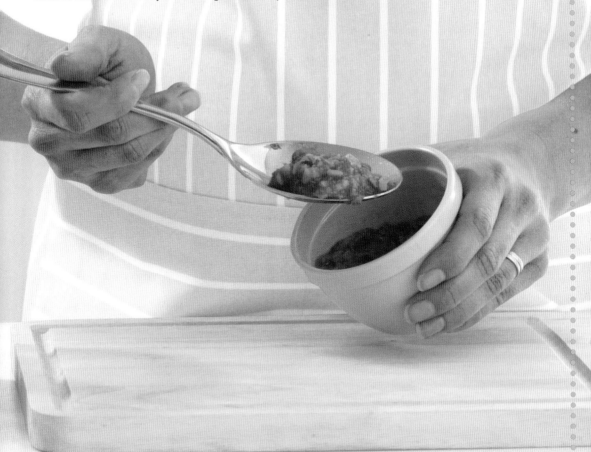

Beef Ragout with Sweet Potato and Apple

Red meat is your baby's best source of iron and she will love it cooked with apple and sweet-tasting root vegetables, such as sweet potato or parsnip. Some babies reject meat because of its texture; however, the sweet potato and apple in this recipe give the meat a nice smooth texture—not to mention a slightly sweet flavor that babies love.

✳ Makes 4 portions ✳ Suitable from 6 months ✳ Prep time 12 minutes ✳ Cooking time 1 hour 25 minutes ✳ Suitable for freezing ✳ Provides protein, carbohydrates, beta-carotene, B vitamins, vitamin C, iron, zinc, fiber

Ingredients:

1 tbsp olive oil
1 small red onion, peeled and chopped
½ celery rib, strings removed (see tip, page 80) and chopped
1 medium carrot, peeled and diced
1 garlic clove, peeled and crushed
4oz lean stewing steak trimmed of fat and cut into small cubes
1 tbsp tomato paste
1 small sweet potato (about 9oz), peeled and diced
1 small dessert apple, peeled and chopped
1½ tsp fresh chopped thyme, or ½ tsp dried thyme
1 cup unsalted chicken or vegetable stock
2 tbsp pure apple juice or water

Method:

1 Preheat the oven to 325°F.

2 Heat the oil in a Dutch oven and sauté the onion, celery, and carrot for 5 minutes, stirring until softened and lightly browned. Add the garlic and sauté for 1 minute, stirring.

3 Gently stir in the cubes of meat and sauté for 2–3 minutes until browned. Stir in the remaining ingredients. Bring to a boil then cover and cook in the oven for 1 hour. Stir halfway through. After 1 hour, remove the lid and continue to cook for another 15 minutes.

4 Purée until smooth in a food processor or place in a bowl and use a hand blender. For older babies, chop in a food processor or by hand to the desired consistency.

5 Freeze in individual portions. When needed, thaw overnight in the refrigerator or for 1–2 hours at room temperature, then microwave or reheat in a small pan until piping hot. Stir and allow to cool before serving.

Apple, Apricot, and Banana Purée

This fresh fruity dessert is a lovely after-dinner treat for little ones, or you can stir it into a little oatmeal for breakfast. Always use ripe bananas, as unripe ones are not easily digested and can cause gas.

✳ Makes 3–4 portions ✳ Suitable from 6 months ✳ Prep time 8 minutes ✳ Cooking time 10 minutes ✳ Suitable for freezing ✳ Provides beta-carotene, potassium, vitamin C, fiber

Ingredients:

2 sweet dessert apples (such as Pink Lady or Gala), peeled, cored, and diced
8 dried apricots, cut into small pieces or snipped with scissors
6–7 tbsp water
1 small banana, sliced

Method:

1 Place the apple and dried apricots into a heavy-bottomed saucepan with 6 tablespoons of the water. Bring to a boil, reduce the heat, cover, and cook gently for about 8 minutes until tender.

2 Add the banana and an extra tablespoon of water, if necessary. Bring back to a boil, reduce the heat, cover, and cook for another 2 minutes.

3 Blend the fruit to a smooth purée in a food processor, or place in a bowl and use a hand blender.

4 Freeze in individual portions. When needed, thaw overnight in the refrigerator or for 1–2 hours at room temperature.

Variation: Creamy Fruit Fool

To boost the calcium content, make a creamy fruit fool by combining 2–3 tablespoons of the Apple, Apricot, and Banana Purée (or any other fruit purées) with 2 tablespoons of thick full-fat vanilla yogurt. Chill until ready to serve.

Apple and Pear with Apricots

The sweet taste and velvety texture of this smooth purée will make it a fast favorite with even the pickiest of eaters.

✳ Makes 4 portions ✳ Suitable from 6 months ✳ Prep time 8 minutes ✳ Cooking time 8 minutes
✳ Suitable for freezing ✳ Provides vitamin A, vitamin C, iron, fiber

Ingredients:

2 sweet dessert apples, peeled, cored, and diced
2 ripe pears, peeled, cored, and diced
8 dried apricots, cut into small pieces
¼ cup water or pure apple juice

Method:

1 Put the fruit into a heavy-bottomed saucepan with the water or pure apple juice. Bring to a boil, reduce the heat, cover, and cook gently for about 8 minutes until tender, adding a little more water or juice if necessary.

2 Blend the fruit to a purée in a food processor or place in a bowl and use a hand blender.

3 Freeze in individual portions. When needed, thaw overnight in the refrigerator or for 1–2 hours at room temperature.

Apple, Pear, and Prune Purée

Prunes are highly nutritious, although some do have tough skins. If your baby won't tolerate the "bits," rub the purée through a fine strainer after blending.

✳ Makes 3 portions ✳ Suitable from 6 months ✳ Prep time 8 minutes ✳ Cooking time 8 minutes
✳ Suitable for freezing ✳ Provides vitamin A, vitamin C, B vitamins, potassium, fiber

Ingredients:

1 sweet dessert apple, peeled, cored, and diced
1 juicy ripe pear, peeled, cored, and diced
6 ready-to-eat prunes, cut into small pieces or
  snipped with scissors
3 tbsp pure apple juice or water

Method:

1 Place the fruit in a saucepan with the pure apple juice or water. Bring to a boil, reduce the heat, cover, and cook gently for 8 minutes until tender, adding a little more water or juice if necessary.

2 Blend the fruit to a purée in a food processor or place in a bowl and use a hand blender.

3 Freeze in individual portions. When needed, thaw overnight in the refrigerator or for 1–2 hours at room temperature.

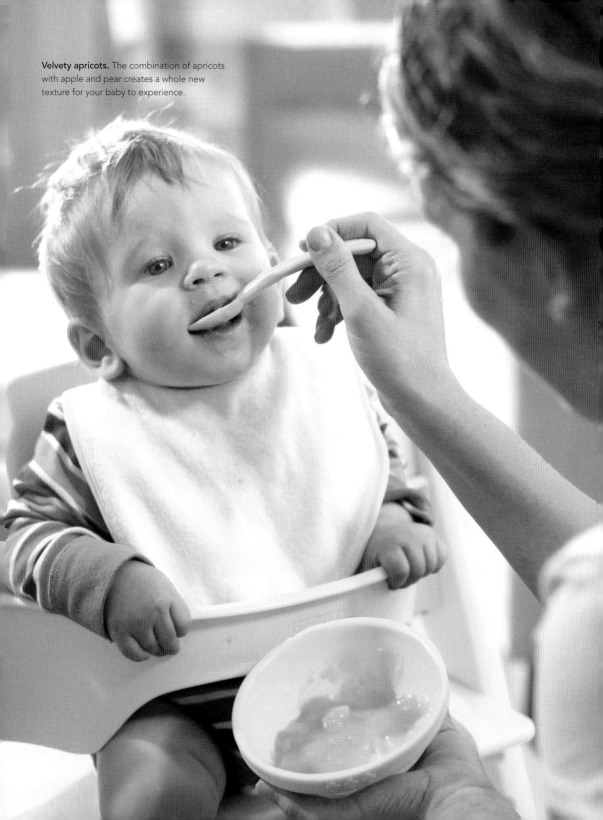

Velvety apricots. The combination of apricots with apple and pear creates a whole new texture for your baby to experience.

Pear and Plum Compôte

The fall-time flavors of this delicious purée are ideal on their own, and also blend well with full-fat yogurt or a little baby rice. Choose plums of any color and size; in fact, the greater the variety, the higher the nutrient value of the purée. If you choose to include the cinnamon, this not only adds a warm rich flavor, but it can encourage healthy digestion.

✱ Makes 3 portions   ✱ Suitable from 6 months   ✱ Prep time 8 minutes   ✱ Cooking time 20–30 minutes
✱ Suitable for freezing   ✱ Provides vitamin A, vitamin C, B vitamins, fiber

Ingredients:
Scant ¼ cup concentrated pure apple juice
2 ripe pears, peeled, cored, and diced
3 large plums, skinned (see tip, page 77), pitted,
   and chopped
Small pinch ground cinnamon (optional)
Few drops natural vanilla extract

Method:
1 Boil the pure apple juice for 3–5 minutes until reduced by half.

2 Place the pears, plums, and cinnamon in a heavy-bottomed saucepan. Cover and cook gently for 5–10 minutes until the juices run from the fruit.

3 Uncover and simmer for 10–20 minutes until the fruit is soft and the liquid has evaporated (the cooking time will depend on the ripeness of the fruit). Stir in the concentrated pure apple juice and the vanilla extract.

4 Mash or purée in a food processor, place in a bowl and use a hand blender, or rub through a strainer.

5 Freeze in individual portions. When required, thaw overnight in the refrigerator or for 1–2 hours at room temperature.

Menu planner: 6 to 9 months

Once your baby is happy eating her first fruit and vegetable purées, you will need to expand her diet to include protein and nutrient-dense foods such as chicken, meat, and cheese to fuel her rapid growth. It's important to include iron in her diet as soon as possible, as stores start to run out after six months. Begin introducing new textures from about seven or eight months.

Day	Breakfast	Lunch	Mid afternoon	Dinner	Bedtime
1	Baby cereal and Apple Purée Breast/bottle	Chicken with Sweet Potato, Peas, and Basil; Banana Purée Breast/bottle	Breast/bottle	Cod with Butternut Squash and Cheese Sauce Breast/bottle	Breast/bottle
2	Baby cereal, Apple and Pear with Apricots; yogurt Breast/bottle	Poached Salmon with Carrots and Peas; Pear and Plum Compôte Breast/bottle	Breast/bottle	Lentil Purée with Sweet Potato Breast/bottle	Breast/bottle
3	Baby cereal and Banana Purée Breast/bottle	Lentil Purée with Sweet Potato; Apple, Pear, and Prune Purée Breast/bottle	Breast/bottle	Chicken with Sweet Potato, Peas, and Basil Breast/bottle	Breast/bottle
4	Grilled cheese on toast fingers Breast/bottle	Beef Ragout with Sweet Potato and Apple; Apple and Pear with Apricots; Breast/bottle	Breast/bottle	Cheesy Leek, Sweet Potato, and Cauliflower Breast/bottle	Breast/bottle
5	Baby cereal and Pear Purée Breast/bottle	Lentil Purée with Sweet Potato; Pear and Plum Compôte Breast/bottle	Breast/bottle	Cod with Butternut Squash and Cheese Sauce Breast/bottle	Breast/bottle
6	Scrambled egg with toast fingers Breast/bottle	Poached Salmon with Carrot and Peas; Mango Purée Breast/bottle	Breast/bottle	Beef Ragout with Sweet Potato and Apple Breast/bottle	Breast/bottle
7	Baby cereal and Apple and Pear with Apricots Breast/bottle	Spinach and Cod Purée; Peach and Banana Purée Breast/bottle	Breast/bottle	Cheesy Leek, Sweet Potato, and Cauliflower Breast/bottle	Breast/bottle

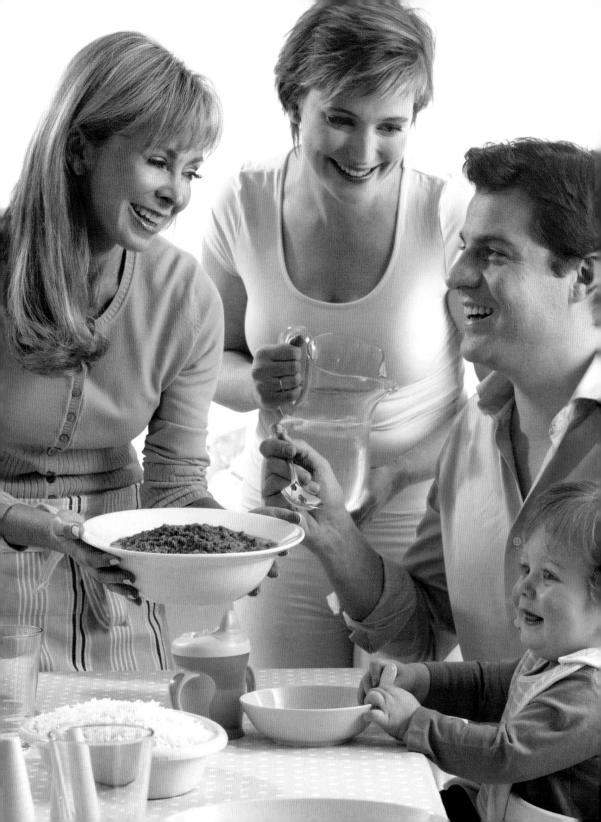

Creating a varied diet

Once your baby is **happy with a variety** of foods and textures, he'll become used to the idea of mealtimes and work toward **eating three meals a day.** As his milk intake decreases, it becomes increasingly important that **his diet is balanced.** You can adjust family meals to make them appropriate for his little tummy, and encourage him to eat along **with the whole family.** It's time, too, for him to start learning to feed himself, so be prepared for a mess!

★ Menu planner page 124

A balanced diet at 10 to 12 months

As your baby heads toward his first birthday, and you begin to give him fewer milk feeds, it does become even more important that his diet is balanced and varied. His tummy is small, so everything he eats should contribute something to his overall nutritional intake.

How to plan your baby's diet

A varied diet includes a variety of different foods. We know that babies need the basics of protein, carbohydrates, fats, and vitamins and minerals (see pages 14–17), and that the best way to make sure that they get what they need is to offer different foods as often as possible. So, you could offer vegetarian proteins such as tofu or legumes at one meal, fish or chicken at the next, and a scrambled egg or yogurt at another. Wheat-based pastas or breads are a good source of carbohydrates, but it's even better to include some alternative forms, such as rice, potatoes, and different grains, such as quinoa, buckwheat, or oats, from time to time. Experiment with the whole spectrum of brightly

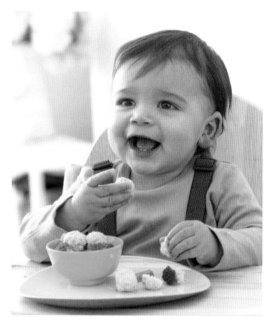

Five a day. Lightly steamed vegetables as a finger food snack help make sure your baby gets his five a day.

The vast majority of babies, left to their own devices, do not overeat, and unless you feed him long past the point that he is willing to eat, you should have no problems.

colored fruits and vegetables, eating sweet potatoes and butternut squash in place of traditional favorites, and offering berries and exotic fruits such as mango, kiwi, and papaya instead of apples and bananas. Go for spring greens, spinach, or even kale, and strips of roasted red pepper, zucchini, or squash for color and key nutrients. The wider the range you can offer your baby, the better.

Creating a balance

You should be aiming to include a carbohydrate, a protein, and a fruit or vegetable at every meal, then adding fruit and vegetables so that you have five servings of these per day. Aim for one iron-rich protein (for example, meat, fish, or poultry) per day and make sure that other meals contain other proteins. Ideally, your baby will be getting fish once or twice a week as well, to make sure he's getting plenty of healthy fats (EFAs). Nut butters, avocados, ground seeds, and fortified eggs and dairy products will also boost his intake of the fats he needs. He doesn't need to eat much of any one food group—aim for lots of variety and you'll get it just right.

Three meals a day

By the end of your baby's first year, he will be eating three meals a day, although the amount of food he eats at each meal can vary considerably. You may want to feed him a little less milk first thing in the morning, so that he finds breakfast easier to manage. You may also decide to offer him milk feeds between or after meals, so that he's hungry enough to eat what's on offer. If he's a grazer, don't worry. Some babies prefer to eat little and often and as long as what you offer is nutritious and balanced, it's fine to operate this way. Remember that the vast majority of babies, left to their own devices, do not overeat, and unless you feed him long past the point that he is willing to eat, you should have no problems.

What can I offer for dessert?

As your baby approaches his first birthday, desserts can certainly feature in his daily diet. They aren't strictly necessary, of course, but they do provide some incentive for finishing off the main course. If he knows there's a "treat" coming up, he'll want to eat up his first course. There's no need to start cooking up special desserts. Fresh-fruit purée mixed with yogurt, a homemade cookie, some dried fruit, or a fresh-fruit ice pop at the end of the meal will make a welcome reward for a job well done.

Healthy snacks

Some babies are hungrier than others, and when a growth spurt is coming up, most are ravenous. You may find that your baby's regular meals and milk feeds simply aren't enough to keep him going. If so, snacks can certainly be on the menu—and they're a wonderful way to include foods or food groups in your baby's diet that he might not easily fit into his normal meals.

Why not create a little snack tray for him with some delicious, nutritious finger foods, such as toast fingers with hummus, berries, chunks of cheese, lightly steamed vegetables, mini sandwiches filled with cheese or tuna, and a mini rice cake. It's important to consider snacks as part of the overall diet, and an extension of your baby's meal times, rather than a "treat."

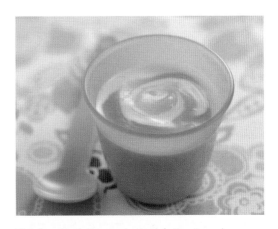

Time for a snack. Yogurt mixed with fruit purée, such as peach, is a healthier choice than ready-flavored yogurt.

Moving on to new textures

Not all babies take kindly to lumps in their food, but most will master a variety of textures if you persevere. While it's perfectly fine to continue to purée some foods for your baby, by 10 to 12 months the time has come for her to learn to chew and swallow. The good news is that there's lots you can do to encourage her to enjoy expanding her food repertoire!

Mashing, grinding, and chopping

Mashing vegetables together, such as potato, carrot, and broccoli with a little butter, milk, and grated cheese, is a good way to introduce different textures. You can also mash well-cooked and raw fruit, and it's a good way to blend several fruits and/or vegetables together without the use of your food processor. Grinding foods will also produce pieces that are whole enough to have a little bite, but soft enough to be chewed and swallowed easily. Once ground and mashed foods are accepted by your little one, try finely cutting and chopping her food, gradually increasing the size of the pieces as she becomes accustomed to the new texture. Some babies actually prefer larger, identifiable lumps to smaller ones that take them by surprise.

> 66 While it's perfectly fine to continue to purée some foods for your baby, the time has come for her to learn to chew and swallow. 99

Meat, poultry, and other proteins

Meat can sometimes be difficult for babies to chew, and this can put them off, so mixing cooked ground meat or chicken with pasta or mashed potatoes is good, or you can make mini meat or chicken balls or mini burgers. Pieces of roast chicken make a good finger food. Alternatively, you can serve up breaded chicken or fish fingers. Tougher cuts of meat such as lamb and beef can be slow-cooked to make them more tender and easier to manage. You could also consider adding tiny pieces of meat to pastas and risottos, where they aren't quite so overwhelming.

Try offering healthy proteins, such as legumes, whole, in the form of finger foods. For example, chickpeas, lima beans, and even kidney beans are usually happily eaten by babies when you serve them this way.

Mixing textures

Create a little plate for your baby that offers foods of all sorts of textures. For example, you could cook some ground chicken balls, mash some potatoes, and offer some raw vegetables, such as carrot or cucumber, with a tasty dip. Or process together some cooked vegetables, such as carrots, zucchini, and sweet pepper with a tomato sauce, and serve with pasta shapes, followed by a homemade cookie or mini muffin.

You can also offer a variety of fruit, vegetables, meat, fish or poultry, dairy, and carbs at the same meal, allowing her to choose some from a tray of finger foods, and feeding her some of the smoother foods from a spoon. She'll end up chewing the finger foods at the same time as she takes in whatever you are offering on the spoon, blending the different flavors and textures. Encourage her to use her finger foods to dip and mush other foods on her plate. She'll be able to create her own concoctions, which will have a texture all of their own. It's good to have a plate or bowl with divisions, as babies like to keep different foods separate.

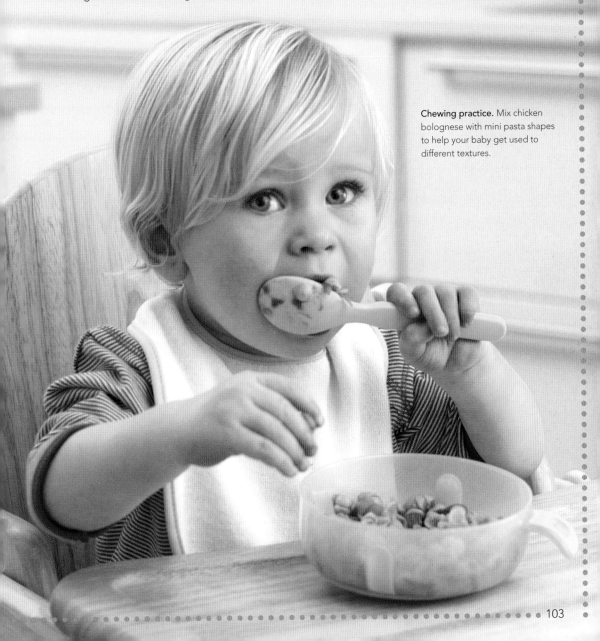

Chewing practice. Mix chicken bolognese with mini pasta shapes to help your baby get used to different textures.

Successful self-feeding

All babies will eventually learn to feed themselves, even if it takes a while to do so successfully. You can, however, encourage the process by allowing your baby to experiment with self-feeding early on. Let him play with his food and make sure you give him plenty of finger foods to suck, gnaw, or actually eat, alongside every meal.

How long does it take?

Most little ones are unable to feed themselves properly before they are at least two or three years old, and until that time, they will rely on mom, dad, or their carer to make sure that the right amount of food makes it into their mouths. Your baby may object to you feeding him if he is feeling particularly independent, and you may have a tussle on your hands as you try to take charge again. You can, however, usually distract him in order to get a little food into his mouth, or help him guide his spoon in the right direction. Try to feed him a good proportion of his meal, so that you know exactly what he's getting. Although some babies can clear a bowl themselves in record time, chances are that most of its contents will end up in their bib, down the sides of their highchair, or scattered all over the floor.

Give your baby a small spoon or soft, flexible fork with a chubby handle that he can grip easily and allow him to scoop the contents of his bowl (or yours!) toward his mouth. Encourage him to pick up finger foods, too. Most things end up in a baby's mouth at this age, so it's a good habit to encourage, as he'll be more likely to try new things if he feels he's in the driving seat.

He'll probably use his hands to eat even the messiest foods for many months to come, so be prepared by using bibs and putting a splash

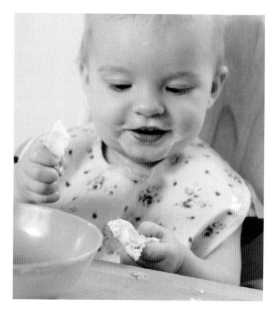

Touch and feel. Enouraging your baby to play with food is a key part of the weaning process, as she learns how to eat.

mat under the high chair so that food that is dropped on the floor can be recycled or more easily cleared up.

Playing with food

This is an important part of the developmental process of learning to eat, so it should be encouraged. The mess may be dispiriting, but your baby should be allowed to touch and feel his food, and to guide it in the direction of his mouth without fear of upsetting you. He'll discover the way the different textures feel and taste, and will be interested in discovering new wonders.

Reluctant self-feeders

Some babies are simply not interested in feeding themselves and rely on you entirely to get food from bowl to mouth. While your baby is still very much dependent at this age and does require regular feeding alongside any self-feeding efforts, it is a good idea to encourage him to try. Why not buy a bright new set of cutlery for him and give him a bowl that's all his own? Present it with a flourish and show him what to do. It's important to remember that babies are not born knowing how to use a spoon or fork, so you can guide his hand at every meal, or show him by doing it yourself, until he gets the hang of it.

> ❝Let him play with his food and give him plenty of finger foods to suck, gnaw, or actually eat, alongside every meal. ❞

You may want to give him a bowl of food at the start of his meal, when he's more hungry, and leave him to it for five minutes or so. Chances are, he'll manage to get at least something into his mouth. Furthermore, babies are great mimics and like nothing better than being like mom and dad, or siblings. Give your baby plenty of opportunity to share mealtimes with the whole family, and he'll soon work out what he's supposed to be doing.

If all the above fail, don't panic. Your baby may just enjoy the process of being fed and will get to grips with the basics later on. Continue to inspire him with delicious meals, and praise his efforts.

David asks . . .

My baby flings his bowl across the room and throws everything on his tray. I have no idea how much he's eating and the mess is driving me crazy!

First of all, you will need to accept that most babies are messy, and eating with their hands, playing with food, and mushing it between their fingers all encourage them to learn about different foods. In my experience, babies who are allowed to play with their food tend to be better eaters, because they enjoy mealtimes, have the opportunity to experiment, and learn to self-feed that much earlier.

Having said that, you can set a few basic ground rules. You can discourage him from throwing food by expressing your disapproval, and taking away his bowl each time he does this. You can also dispense with the bowl for the time being, placing his food directly on his tray, or investing in a bowl with a suction cup at the base to prevent it from being lifted.

You may also want to consider whether he's a little bored when he starts throwing his food around. Maybe he's actually had enough and is itching to be released from his highchair.

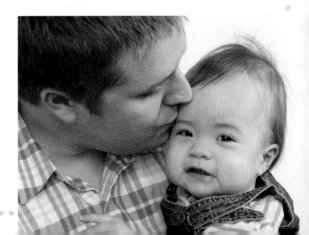

Family food

One of the best parts of introducing your baby to a greater variety of tastes and textures is that she can become involved in family meals. Some recipes must be adjusted to make sure your baby isn't having too much sugar or salt, but this can make the whole family more aware of what's in their food.

Adapting family meals

Most whole, fresh foods are appropriate for babies and you'll simply need to be sure that you don't add salt or sugar (watch the condiments and cooking sauces, too). So, roasting a chicken, mashing some potatoes, and serving up some creamed spinach and baby carrots will provide the perfect meal for a little one. Finely chop, mash, or even purée the chicken and carrots and your child's meal is ready without further cooking. Similarly, you can process family soups, stews, casseroles, and even pasta dishes in your food processor for a moment or two, perhaps adding a little extra liquid to make it easier for your baby to manage.

Sharing mealtimes helps to create healthy, positive associations with food, as your baby learns to enjoy the social experience.

What about herbs and spices?

There are no specific spices or herbs that need to be off the menu for babies (apart from salt and sugar), but some babies simply do not like the taste of some flavorings and others may have their tummies upset by them. It's a good idea to try one new flavoring at a time, and if there appears to be no problem, you can move on to try whatever your baby likes.

Herbs are a delicious and nutritious addition to baby foods and can spice up, or make more fragrant, foods that might otherwise seem a little flavorless. Any of the green herbs, such as cilantro, basil, thyme, parsley, and dill, can be added easily, and you can use cinnamon, rosemary, and bay leaves while cooking fish, chicken, or vegetables. The more flavors to which your little one becomes accustomed while she's small, the wider the variety of "likes" that will be established.

If your baby likes the flavors and has no reactions after eating them (watch for diarrhea, crying, rashes, and drawn-up knees), then you can introduce whatever spices appeal. In some cultures, babies are brought up on strong, spicy foods and cope very well. So experiment to see what your baby will enjoy.

The importance of eating together

Sharing mealtimes helps to create healthy, positive associations with food, as your baby learns to enjoy the social experience. Studies show that children who eat with their parents are more likely to consume more fruits and vegetables and eat fewer fatty and sugary foods. The reason is that they develop good habits based on the family ethos and also eat a wider range of foods, which they will try because everyone is eating them. Most babies love to copy parents and siblings, so offer your baby a little of your food and you'll be amazed by what she will eat.

Out and about

While it's a good idea to stay at home when you first start the weaning process, the time will quickly arrive when you'll need to feed your baby while you are out and about. You may also need to prepare meals for her to eat at daycare or at the babysitter's.

Transporting your baby's food

A good cool bag, with an ice pack, should keep your baby's purées at the right temperature. If you need to keep a purée chilled for a long period of time, you could invest in a wide-necked thermos into which you can place some chilled purée or several frozen purée cubes. Make sure you heat the purée until piping hot and then let it cool before serving to destroy any bacteria.

Many finger foods are easy to transport, and will last a few hours at room temperature. Fruit and vegetables, bread fingers, mini sandwiches, rice cakes, and dried fruits will all keep your baby's tummy full, no matter where you are. You can also choose foods that can be puréed, mashed, or cut into chunks on the spot, such as bananas, mango, papaya, or very ripe pears or peaches.

Your baby's lunchbox

You may wish to prepare a lunchbox for your baby, when she goes to daycare or the babysitter, or if you are taking her out for the day. You can create a healthy, delicious meal from finger foods, including mini cheeses, pieces of chicken or mini chicken balls, mini sandwiches with cream cheese, or cucumber and carrot sticks wrapped in damp paper towels to keep them fresh. For dessert, take fresh and dried fruits or containers of fruit purée, yogurt, or fromage frais. Bananas are ideal as they come in their own packaging, and slices of mango, dried or fresh, are also good choices.

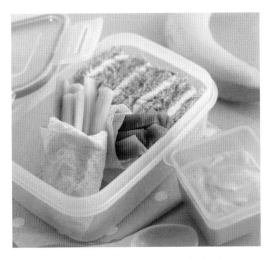

A taste of home. When you are heading out for the day, create a delicious lunchbox from your baby's favorite finger foods.

If you want to give your baby a hot meal while you are out, such as a purée or a pasta dish with small pasta shapes, heat the food to a high temperature at home and decant it instantly into a thermos designed to keep it hot for up to four hours.

Eating out

Babies can be adventurous eaters and will happily pick at things from your plate. You could encourage her to try plain pasta, fresh bread, fruits or veggies, mashed potatoes, mashed eggs, well-cooked rice mashed to a purée with milk, and fresh, ripe fruits, crushed until smooth. You can also offer your baby tastes of sauces that you may be eating.

Tomato and Basil Pasta Sauce

Stirring in fresh basil and Parmesan is a good way to add flavor, because you don't want to season this delicious creamy tomato sauce with salt. You can freeze the sauce on its own in individual portions then reheat and add to freshly cooked pasta before serving if you prefer, or use to serve with other recipes in this book, such as Cheesy Rice Balls (see page 114), Cherub's Couscous (see opposite), or Mini meatballs (see page 116).

✹ Makes 4 portions ✹ Suitable from 10 months ✹ Prep time 5 minutes ✹ Cooking time 20 minutes
✹ Suitable for freezing ✹ Provides protein, beta-carotene, vitamin D, vitamin C, calcium, fiber
(and carbohydrates when served with pasta)

Ingredients:
1 tbsp olive oil
½ small onion, peeled and chopped
½ garlic clove, peeled and crushed
1 small carrot, peeled and shredded
Scant 1 cup puréed tomatoes
3 tbsp water
2 fresh basil leaves, coarsely chopped
1 tsp freshly shredded Parmesan cheese
1 tbsp full-fat cream cheese

To serve:
½ cup conchigliette (baby pasta shells)

Method:
1 Heat the oil in a saucepan. Add the onion, garlic, and carrot, then stir, cover, and cook gently for 5 minutes to soften.

2 Add the tomatoes and water. Bring to a boil, reduce the heat, cover, and simmer gently for 15 minutes.

3 Purée the sauce with the basil and cheeses in a food processor or place in a bowl and use a hand blender.

4 Meanwhile, cook the pasta shells in boiling water according to package directions. Drain and return to the pan. Stir in the sauce, cool slightly, and serve.

5 Freeze in individual portions. When needed, thaw overnight in the refrigerator or for 1–2 hours at room temperature, then microwave or reheat in a small pan until piping hot. Stir and allow to cool before serving.

Cherub's Couscous

If your baby likes moist textures, mix this with a little Tomato and Basil Pasta Sauce (see opposite) or a spoonful of warm puréed tomatoes before serving.

✳ Makes 3–4 portions ✳ Suitable from 10 months ✳ Prep time 10 minutes ✳ Cooking time 15 minutes ✳ Suitable for freezing ✳ Provides protein, carbohydrates, beta-carotene, vitamin C, B vitamins, calcium, iron, zinc, fiber

Ingredients:
2 tsp olive oil
½ small onion, peeled and chopped
¼ orange bell pepper, seeded and chopped
1 small chicken breast, cut into small cubes
½ garlic clove, peeled and crushed
2 tbsp frozen peas
6 tbsp unsalted fresh chicken or vegetable stock
   or water
Generous ⅓ cup quick cooking couscous
2 tbsp freshly shredded Parmesan cheese

Method:
1 Heat the oil in a saucepan and sauté the onion, bell pepper, and chicken gently for 3 minutes, stirring. Stir in the garlic and sauté for 30 seconds.

2 Add the peas and stock or water, bring to a boil, reduce the heat, cover, and simmer gently for 5 minutes or until the chicken and vegetables are tender.

3 Stir in the couscous, remove from the heat, cover, and let stand for 5 minutes (or as the package directs). Fluff the couscous with a fork and mix in the Parmesan before serving.

4 Freeze in individual portions. When needed, thaw overnight in the refrigerator or for 1–2 hours at room temperature, then microwave or reheat in a small pan until piping hot. Stir and allow to cool before serving.

Pasta "Risotto"

This delicious dish is bursting with flavor. You can add extra vegetables if you like, such as corn and broccoli, to provide even more nutrients.

✳ Makes 4 portions ✳ Suitable from 10 months ✳ Prep time 5 minutes ✳ Cooking time 11 minutes
✳ Suitable for freezing ✳ Provides carbohydrates, protein, beta-carotene, folic acid, vitamin C, calcium, fiber

Ingredients:
⅔ cup orzo or other small pasta shapes
1 small carrot, peeled and cut into very small dice
1 cup boiling water
1 small zucchini, peeled and cut into very
   small dice
3 tbsp frozen peas
1 tbsp unsalted butter, cut into small flakes
¼ cup freshly shredded Parmesan cheese

Method:
1 Put the pasta in a saucepan together with the carrot. Cover with the boiling water, bring back to a boil, stir, reduce the heat, cover, and simmer gently for 5 minutes.

2 Add the zucchini, re-cover, and cook for 3 minutes. Stir in the peas and cook for another 3 minutes.

3 Stir in the butter and Parmesan. Cool slightly before serving.

4 Freeze in individual portions. When needed, thaw overnight in the refrigerator or for 1–2 hours at room temperature, then microwave or reheat in a small pan until piping hot. Stir and allow to cool before serving.

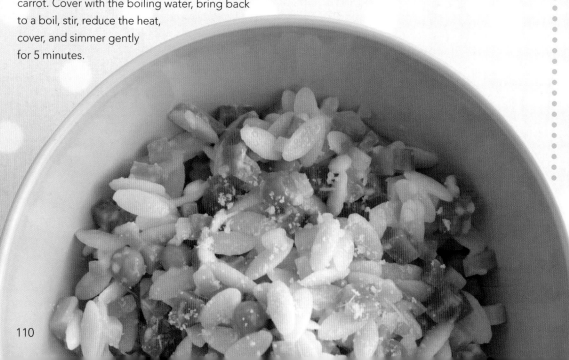

Chicken Bolognese

This flavorful dish is a delicious alternative to traditional Bolognese sauce and it works well with any type of pasta. Rich in protein, beta-carotene, antioxidants, and even a little iron, it is a balanced meal in a bowl. You can freeze the sauce separately in individual portions if you like, then serve with freshly cooked pasta, rice, or potatoes.

✷ Makes 4 portions ✷ Suitable from 10 months ✷ Prep time 10 minutes ✷ Cooking time 15 minutes
✷ Suitable for freezing ✷ Provides protein, beta-carotene, vitamin C, B vitamins, iron, zinc (and carbohydrates when served with pasta, rice, or potatoes)

Ingredients:

1 tbsp olive oil
½ small onion, peeled and finely chopped
1 small carrot, peeled and shredded
½ large or 1 small garlic clove, peeled and crushed
⅓ cup ground chicken (I use thigh meat)
½ tsp fresh chopped thyme, or good pinch
    dried thyme
Scant 1 cup puréed tomatoes
Scant ½ cup pure apple juice
1 tsp tomato paste
½ tsp Worcestershire sauce
4 fresh basil leaves, chopped

To serve:
½ cup conchigliette (baby pasta shells)

Method:

1 Heat the oil in a saucepan and sauté the onion and carrot gently, stirring, for 3 minutes to soften. Add the garlic and sauté for another 30 seconds.

2 Add the ground chicken and sauté, stirring, until it turns opaque and all the grains are separate.

3 Add the thyme, tomatoes, and apple juice. Bring to a boil and stir in the tomato paste and Worcestershire sauce. Reduce the heat, cover, and simmer gently for 10 minutes. Stir in the basil.

4 Meanwhile, cook the pasta shells in boiling water according to package directions. Drain and return to the pan. Stir in the sauce, cool slightly, and serve.

5 Freeze in individual portions. When needed, thaw overnight in the refrigerator or for 1–2 hours at room temperature, then microwave or reheat in a small pan until piping hot. Stir and allow to cool before serving.

Annabel's Tasty Bolognese

Red meat provides the best source of iron for your baby, which is particularly important between six months and two years. The sautéed red onion, carrot, and apple add a delicious flavor to this sauce. You can freeze the sauce on its own in individual portions then reheat and serve with freshly cooked pasta, rice, or mashed potatoes if you prefer.

🌟 Makes 4 portions 🌟 Suitable from 10 months 🌟 Prep time 10 minutes 🌟 Cooking time 30 minutes 🌟 Suitable for freezing 🌟 Provides protein, beta-carotene, vitamin C, iron, zinc, fiber (and carbohydrates when served with pasta, rice, or potatoes)

Ingredients:

1 tbsp sunflower oil
1 small red onion, peeled and finely chopped
1 small carrot, peeled and shredded
½ celery rib, strings removed (see tip, page 80) and finely chopped
½ small dessert apple, shredded
4 tbsp water
Scant 1 cup puréed tomatoes
Scant ¾ cup lean ground beef
1 small garlic clove, peeled and crushed
¼ cup unsalted fresh beef or vegetable stock or water
1 tsp fresh chopped thyme, or ¼ tsp dried thyme

To serve:

½ cup conchigliette (baby pasta shells)

Method:

1 Heat the oil in a saucepan and gently sauté the onion, carrot, celery, and apple for 2 minutes. Add the water, stir, cover, and cook very gently for 8 minutes until soft.

2 Transfer the vegetables to a food processor, add the tomatoes, and process until blended.

3 Meanwhile, dry-fry the ground beef in a non-stick frying pan until browned. Add the garlic and sauté for 30 seconds.

4 Pour the tomato and vegetable sauce over the meat. Add the stock or water and the thyme, bring to a boil, reduce the heat, cover, and simmer gently for about 15 minutes until rich and tender.

5 Meanwhile, cook the pasta shells in boiling water according to package directions. Drain and return to the pan. Stir in the sauce, cool slightly, and serve.

6 Freeze in individual portions. When required, thaw overnight in the refrigerator or for 1–2 hours at room temperature, then microwave or reheat in a small pan until piping hot. Stir and allow to cool before serving.

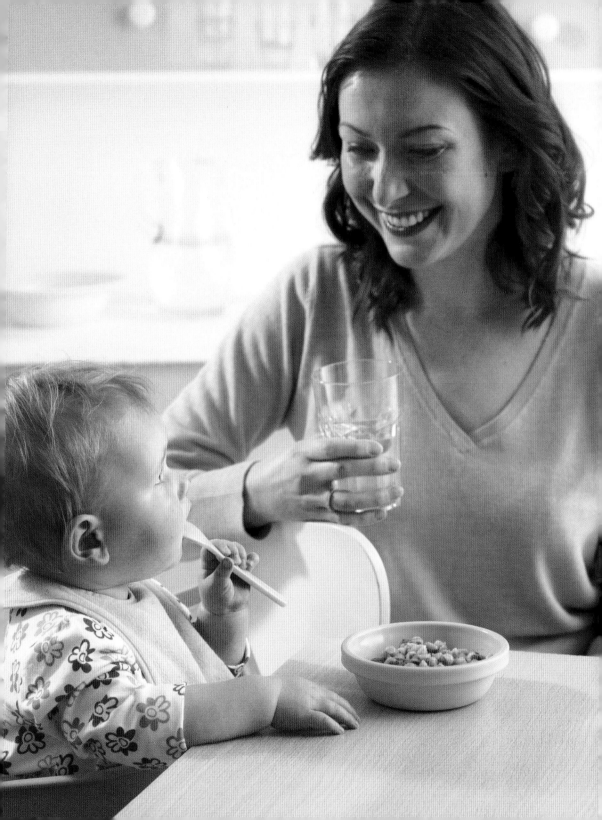

Cheesy Rice Balls

You could serve these with Mini Meatballs (see page 116) or Annabel's Chicken Burgers (opposite) or with carrot, cucumber, or sweet pepper sticks. They are also good served with the Tomato and Basil Pasta Sauce (see page 108) as a dipping sauce.

✳ Makes 22 balls, 5–6 portions ✳ Suitable from 10 months ✳ Prep time 5 minutes ✳ Cooking time 20 minutes ✳ Suitable for freezing ✳ Provides carbohydrates, B vitamins, vitamin D, calcium, protein, fiber

Ingredients:

Scant ½ cup risotto rice
1 cup unsalted vegetable stock or water
½ cup shredded Monterey Jack or Cheddar cheese
2 tbsp freshly shredded Parmesan cheese
2 tsp finely chopped chives
Pepper, to taste

Method:

1 Put the rice and stock or water in a small non-stick saucepan and bring to a boil. Reduce the heat as low as possible, cover, and simmer gently for 10 minutes.

2 Add 2 tablespoons water, stir, re-cover, and cook for another 10 minutes until the stock has been absorbed and the rice is tender.

3 Remove from the heat and leave to stand for 5 minutes, then transfer to a bowl and leave for 10–15 minutes until cool enough to handle. Stir in the cheeses, chives, and season with pepper to taste.

4 Roll teaspoonfuls into balls using your hands. Serve right away, or place in a sealed container and chill immediately. The balls will keep in the refrigerator for 24 hours or can be frozen then thawed overnight in the refrigerator, not at room temperature.

Annabel's Chicken Burgers

These soft, tasty burgers are bound to be a hit with your child—serve with steamed vegetables, such as carrots or broccoli, for a perfect balanced meal.

✦ Makes 12 mini burgers, 4 portions ✦ Suitable from 10 months ✦ Prep time 10 minutes
✦ Cooking time 10 minutes ✦ Suitable for freezing ✦ Provides protein, vitamin C, calcium, iron, zinc, fiber

Ingredients:

1 tbsp olive oil
½ small onion, peeled and finely chopped
1 small garlic clove, peeled and crushed
1 cup ground chicken (mix of breast and
  thigh meat)
4 fresh sage leaves, chopped
¼ dessert apple, peeled and shredded
⅓ cup fresh breadcrumbs (1 medium slice bread)
3 tbsp freshly shredded Parmesan cheese
Vegetable oil, for cooking

Method:

1 Heat the olive oil in a small pan and sauté the onion and garlic gently, stirring, for 2 minutes. Allow to cool.

2 In a bowl, mix the ground chicken with the sage, apple, and breadcrumbs. Stir in the cooled onion and garlic and the Parmesan.

3 Using your hands, shape the mixture into 12 small patties.

4 Heat a little vegetable oil in a frying pan and brown the burgers for 1–2 minutes each side. Turn the heat down to low and cook gently for about 5 minutes until cooked through. To test, press the point of a knife down through the center of one of the burgers. Hold for 5 seconds and remove. The blade should feel burning hot. If not, cook a little longer. Drain on paper towels.

Tip:

To freeze, place the burgers (either before or after cooking) on a baking sheet lined with plastic wrap, cover with a second sheet of plastic wrap, and freeze for 2–3 hours until solid. Pack in a rigid container or a sealed plastic bag. Defrost overnight in the refrigerator or for 2–3 hours at room temperature before cooking.

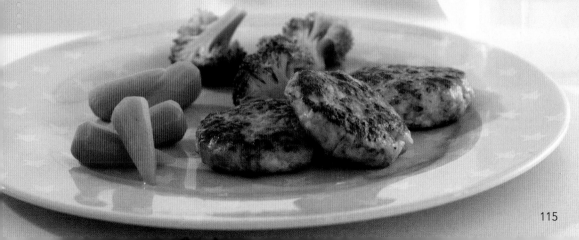

Mini Meatballs

These are also delicious served with Tomato and Basil Pasta Sauce (see page 108), or with steamed vegetables, such as carrots or broccoli.

✿ Makes 25 mini balls, 6–8 portions ✿ Suitable from 10 months ✿ Prep time 15 minutes
✿ Cooking time 6 minutes ✿ Suitable for freezing ✿ Provides protein, vitamin C, calcium, iron, zinc

Ingredients:
2 tsp olive oil
1 medium onion, peeled and finely chopped
1 garlic clove, peeled and crushed
Scant 1 cup lean ground beef
¾ cup fresh white breadcrumbs (2 medium
    slices bread)
1 tbsp chopped fresh parsley
2 tbsp freshly shredded Parmesan cheese
1 tsp tomato paste
½ small dessert apple, peeled and shredded
¼ unsalted vegetable bouillon cube, crumbled
1 egg, beaten
Vegetable oil, for frying

Method:
1 Heat the oil in a saucepan and sauté the onion for 3 minutes, stirring, until softened. Add the garlic and sauté for 30 seconds. Set aside to cool.

2 Mix together the ground beef, breadcrumbs, parsley, Parmesan, tomato paste, apple, and bouillon cube. Stir in the sautéed onion and garlic, and add the beaten egg to bind.

3 Form the mixture into 25 mini meatballs. Heat the oil in a frying pan and sauté the meatballs until browned and cooked inside. Drain on paper towels.

Tip:
To freeze, follow the instructions for freezing Annabel's Chicken Burgers on page 115.

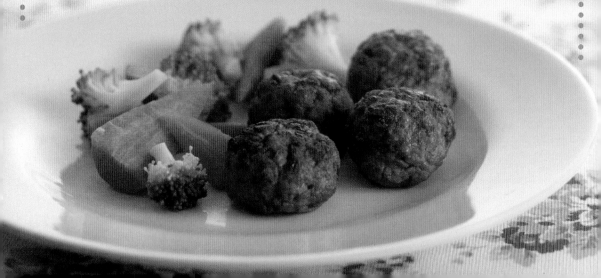

Fish Fingers

These delicious, golden fish fingers can be served to the whole family, and provide plenty of good-quality protein. If you choose white-skinned fillets, there is no need to remove the skin. However, darker-skinned fillets should have their tougher skins removed before preparing.

✸ Makes 6–8 fingers, 3–4 portions ✸ Suitable from 10 months ✸ Prep time 10 minutes
✸ Cooking time 4 minutes ✸ Suitable for freezing, uncooked ✸ Provides protein, calcium, iron

Ingredients:
Generous 1 cup fresh white breadcrumbs
   (3 medium slices bread)
3 tbsp freshly shredded Parmesan cheese
2 tbsp coarsely chopped parsley
Good pinch of paprika (optional)
2 fresh (not frozen) flat white boneless fish fillets
   (e.g., sole, flounder), about 3½oz each, skinned
   (see above)
2 tbsp all-purpose flour
1 egg beaten with 1 tbsp water
Vegetable oil for frying

Method:
1 Put the breadcrumbs, Parmesan, parsley, and paprika (if using) in a food processor and process together until the parsley is finely chopped. Transfer to a large plate.

2 Cut the fish fillets in half lengthwise then into strips the size of little fingers.

3 Put the flour on a plate, and put the beaten egg and water in a shallow dish. Toss each piece of fish in the flour to dust, then dip in the egg, then roll in the breadcrumbs to coat. If you are not cooking immediately, put the coated fish on a baking sheet lined with plastic wrap, cover with a second sheet of plastic wrap, and freeze for 2–3 hours until solid. When frozen, transfer to a rigid container or sealed plastic bag and store in the freezer.

4 To cook, heat a thin layer of oil in a frying pan. Cook fresh or from frozen for about 2–3 minutes each side until golden and cooked through. Drain on paper towels before serving.

Mini Sandwiches to Share

Sandwiches are quick and easy to prepare and make good finger food for your baby. When friends bring their babies around for a visit, you can make a variety of different flavors—and offer them to hungry moms or dads as well. For young babies, it may be better to cut off the crusts from the bread and then flatten the sandwich with a rolling pin.

Banana, Cream Cheese, and Raspberry

✴ Suitable from 10 months ✴ Provides protein, carbohydrates, vitamin C, vitamin D, calcium, potassium, iron, fiber

2 tsp full-fat cream cheese
2 slices bread
½ small banana, mashed
2 tsp low-sugar jam such as apricot

Spread the cream cheese over one slice of bread and spread the mashed banana over the cream cheese. Spread the jam over the second slice of bread and sandwich the two slices together. Cut into 8 small squares.

Other good fillings ...

✴ Shredded cheese
✴ Cream cheese and chopped, dried apricots
✴ Chopped hard-boiled egg mixed with a little mayonnaise and snipped chives
✴ Chopped chicken with mayonnaise
✴ Mashed sardines with a little ketchup
✴ Mashed banana

Tuna or Salmon Mayonnaise

✴ Suitable from 10 months ✴ Provides protein, carbohydrates, vitamin C, vitamin D, EFAs

2 tbsp drained canned tuna or salmon, flaked
2 tsp mayonnaise
1 tsp ketchup
2 slices bread

Mash together the tuna or salmon with the mayonnaise and ketchup. Spread over one slice of bread and sandwich together with the second slice. Cut into 8 small squares.

Tip:

Only use commercial mayonnaise made with processed egg, rather than mayonnaise made with raw egg. Alternatively, use a little Greek yogurt instead.

French Bread Mini Pizza

Babies love joining in at mealtimes, and these pizzas can be adapted for the whole family. You could also use toasted, split English muffins as pizza bases.

✳ Makes 1–2 portions ✳ Suitable from 10 months ✳ Prep time 5 minutes ✳ Cooking time 5 minutes
✳ Provides carbohydrates, protein, vitamin A, vitamin C, vitamin D, B vitamins, calcium

Ingredients:
4 slices from a small baguette or 2 slices about
   ¼in thick from a large baguette
4 generous teaspoons Tomato and Basil Pasta
   Sauce (see page 108) or puréed tomatoes
2–3 fresh basil leaves, chopped (optional)
3 tbsp shredded Cheddar or Mozzarella cheese

Method:
1 Preheat the broiler to high. Toast the bread on both sides under the broiler.

2 Spread the Tomato and Basil Pasta Sauce or tomatoes over the toast. Sprinkle with the basil, if using. Sprinkle the cheese over the top and broil for about 1 minute until the cheese is bubbling.

3 Leave to cool for 1–2 minutes, then cut in half (small baguette) or into 4 pieces (large) to serve.

Cheese and Apple Quesadilla

Quesadillas can be made with lots of different ingredients. Why not try chopped tomatoes or mashed tuna with shredded cucumber in place of apple?

✳ Makes 1 portion ✳ Suitable from 10 months ✳ Prep time 5 minutes ✳ Cooking time 3 minutes
✳ Provides carbohydrates, protein, vitamin C, vitamin D, calcium, fiber

Ingredients:
3 tbsp shredded Monterey Jack or Cheddar cheese
1 small flour tortilla
½ small dessert apple, shredded

Method:
1 Sprinkle the cheese over one half of the tortilla, top with the shredded apple, and fold the other half over.

2 Heat a heavy-bottomed, non-stick frying pan over medium heat. Dry-fry the tortilla for about 1½ minutes, pressing down with a spatula until lightly toasted underneath and the cheese is beginning to melt. Flip over and cook the other side for another 1½ minutes.

3 Leave to cool for 3–4 minutes, then cut into 4 wedges before serving.

Tropical Banana Popsicle

Popsicles are great for babies to suck on when they are teething. You could also make this popsicle using orange juice instead of tropical fruit juice.

✹ Makes 3–4 popsicles ✹ Suitable from 10 months ✹ Prep time 5 minutes
✹ Provides protein, beta-carotene, vitamin C, vitamin D, calcium, fiber

Ingredients:
½ small ripe banana
4½oz tub creamy vanilla full-fat yogurt
Scant ½ cup tropical fruit juice
1 tbsp confectioners' sugar or agave or maple
  syrup (optional)

Method:
1 Blend the banana and yogurt until smooth in a food processor or place in a bowl and use a hand blender.

2 Add the fruit juice and sugar or syrup, if using, and blend until combined. Pour into molds and freeze for several hours or overnight.

Blueberry and Banana Popsicle

Bursting with vitamins and minerals, these deliciously fresh popsicles are a perfect way to make sure your baby gets the nutrients she needs. Blueberries can be swapped for any other berry in season, or why not try a blend?

✹ Makes 4–5 popsicles ✹ Suitable from 10 months ✹ Prep time 5 minutes
✹ Provides protein, vitamin C, vitamin E , potassium, fiber

Ingredients:
⅔ cup blueberries
6 tbsp creamy blueberry full-fat yogurt
¼ ripe banana
1 tbsp confectioners' sugar or agave or maple
  syrup (optional)

Method:
1 Blend the ingredients together until smooth in a food processor or use a hand blender.

2 Rub through a strainer to remove the seeds and skins (if preferred, but not absolutely necessary). Pour into molds and freeze overnight.

Tip:
If you don't have ice popsicle containers, you can freeze the mixture in the sections of an ice-cube tray and stand a piece of plastic drinking straw up in the center of each for the "stick." Each mixture will make between 12 and 18 cubes.

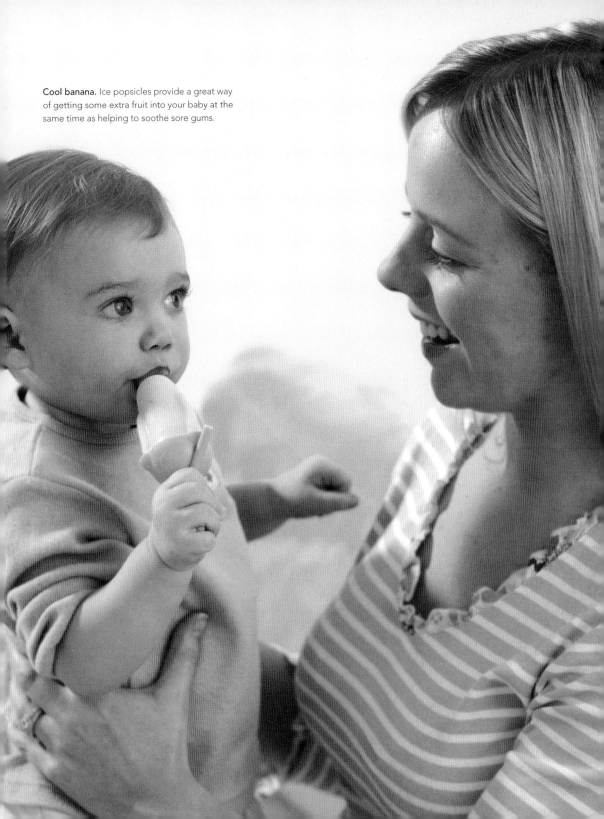

Cool banana. Ice popsicles provide a great way of getting some extra fruit into your baby at the same time as helping to soothe sore gums.

Banana Muffins

If you don't have muffin pans, use double thickness cupcake papers on a baking sheet. Just remove the outer paper after cooling, and reuse next time.

⭐ Makes about 20 mini or 8 standard muffins ⭐ Suitable from 10 months ⭐ Prep time 10 minutes
⭐ Cooking time 12–18 minutes ⭐ Suitable for freezing ⭐ Provides carbohydrates, vitamin C, potassium, iron, fiber

Ingredients:
¼ cup unsalted butter, softened
Scant ½ cup superfine sugar
1 egg
2 small ripe bananas, mashed
½ tsp natural vanilla extract
Generous 1 cup all-purpose flour
1 tsp baking powder
¼ tsp baking soda
¼ tsp salt (optional)
⅓ cup chopped raisins

Method:
1 Preheat the oven to 350°F. Line mini muffin pans with 24 mini cupcake papers, or standard pans with 8 standard cupcake papers.

2 With an electric mixer, beat the butter and sugar until pale, soft, and fluffy. Add the egg, bananas, and vanilla, and beat for 1 minute—the mixture will look a little curdled, but don't worry.

3 Sift together the flour, baking powder, baking soda, and salt, if using. Add to the banana mixture and beat until just combined. Stir in the raisins.

4 Using a 1-ounce ice cream scoop, divide the batter between the cupcake papers and bake for 12–14 minutes for mini ones, 16–18 minutes for larger ones, until golden, risen, and firm to the touch. Cool for 5 minutes, then transfer to a wire rack to cool completely. Store in an airtight container. Alternatively, freeze in a rigid container.

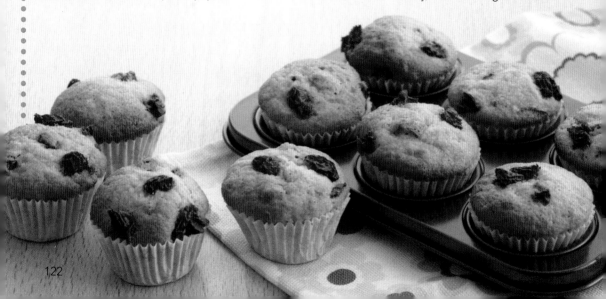

Oat Cookies

These little cookies can be offered as a sweet treat at the end of a meal, and they also work well as a healthy snack. The maple syrup gives them a delightful flavor, while the oats provide a good source of fiber, protein, and B vitamins.

★ Makes 24 small or 12 large cookies ★ Suitable from 10 months ★ Prep time 15 minutes
★ Cooking time 12–18 minutes ★ Provides carbohydrates, protein, B vitamins, iron, fiber

Ingredients:
Generous ½ cup whole-wheat flour
½ cup rolled oats
¼ tsp baking soda
½ cup unsalted softened butter
Generous ¼ cup superfine sugar
1 tbsp maple syrup
1 tsp natural vanilla extract
½ cup raisins or chopped dried apricots

Method:
1 Preheat the oven to 350°F. Put all the ingredients except the fruit in a food processor and pulse for about 1 minute until the mixture forms large clumps of dough. Add the dried fruit to the mixture and pulse briefly to combine.

2 Roll heaped teaspoonfuls of the dough into 24 walnut-sized balls and arrange on two parchment-lined baking sheets. Flatten to a ¼in thickness with the back of a wet spoon. Alternatively, use tablespoonfuls of the mixture to make larger cookies.

3 Bake in the oven for 12–14 minutes for small cookies, 15 minutes for large, until golden.

4 Leave to cool for a few minutes on the baking sheets, then transfer the cookies to a wire rack to cool completely. Store in an airtight container.

Menu planner: 10 to 12 months

I have tried to show variety in my menu planners, but it is also fine to prepare food in batches and freeze, then repeat the same recipes two or three times a week. By 10 months, you can slowly start reducing milk feeds.

Day	Breakfast	Lunch	Mid afternoon	Dinner	Bedtime
1	Cereal; piece of fruit Breast/bottle	Annabel's Chicken Burgers with carrot and broccoli, rice; piece of fruit Breast/bottle	Breast/bottle	Tomato and Basil Sauce with Pasta; yogurt; juice	Breast/bottle
2	Oatmeal and yogurt; piece of fruit Breast/bottle	Annabel's Tasty Bolognese; Oat Cookie; piece of fruit Breast/bottle	Breast/bottle	Fish Fingers with carrot and broccoli, rice; juice	Breast/bottle
3	Scrambled eggs, toast fingers; piece of fruit Breast/bottle	French Bread Mini Pizza; Blueberry and Banana Popsicle Breast/bottle	Breast/bottle	Chicken Bolognese; piece of fruit; juice	Breast/bottle
4	Cereal; piece of fruit Breast/bottle	Mini Meatballs, boiled baby potatoes cut in half, carrot sticks; Oat Cookie Breast/bottle	Breast/bottle	Cheese and Apple Quesadilla, carrot and cucumber sticks; piece of fruit; juice	Breast/bottle
5	Banana Muffin; yogurt; piece of fruit Breast/bottle	Mini Sandwiches, cucumber and carrot sticks; piece of fruit; Oat Cookie Breast/bottle	Breast/bottle	Annabel's Chicken Burger, corn, carrots, and peas; Tropical Banana Popsicle; juice	Breast/bottle
6	Scrambled eggs, toast fingers; piece of fruit Breast/bottle	Fish Fingers with oven-baked potato; yogurt Breast/bottle	Breast/bottle	Mini Meatballs and Pasta "Risotto"; yogurt; juice	Breast/bottle
7	Toast fingers and sticks of cheese; piece of fruit Breast/bottle	Chicken Bolognese; yogurt; piece of fruit Breast/bottle	Breast/bottle	Fish Fingers with carrot and broccoli; Tropical Banana Popsicle; Juice	Breast/bottle

Resources

Annabel Karmel
www.annabelkarmel.com
The top destination for recipes, books, and advice on weaning, feeding children, and family food from Annabel Karmel. See her Make it Easy feeding and food preparation range.

akTV
http://annabelkarmel.tv
The Annabel Karmel online internet TV channel with step-by-step videos of recipes, advice, and top tips.

American Academy of Pediatrics
www.aap.org

BabyCenter
www.babycenter.com

Gerber
www.gerber.com

Parenting
www.parenting.com

Allergy

The Food Allergy Network
www.foodallergy.org

National Institutes of Health
www.nih.gov

Breastfeeding

Breastfeeding.com
www.breastfeeding.com

La Leche League
www.llli.org

National Alliance for Breastfeeding Advocacy
www.naba-breastfeeding.org

Equipment

Amazon
www.amazon.com

Babies R Us
www.babiesrus.com

Target
www.target.com

Nutrition and health

American Heart Association
www.americanheart.org

GoVeg.com
www.goveg.com

Kids Health
www.kidshealth.org

Nutrition.gov
www.nutrition.gov

USDA (Food Pyramid)
www.mypyramid.gov

The Vegetarian Resource Group
www.vrg.org

Index

Index

About the author

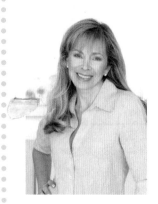

Annabel Karmel is one of the world's most successful writers on children's food and nutrition and her books are published all over the world. An unrivaled expert on all aspects of feeding babies, she offers practical advice on healthy eating and explains how nutritional needs change as a young child grows.

A frequent television guest, el has appeared on *Regis & Kelly*, *The View*, and *The To show*. She has sold more than four million copies of her books worldwide, including *First Meals*, *Mom and Me Cookbook*, *You Can Cook*, *First Meals Food Diary*, and *First Meals & More: Your Questions Answered*.

In 2006, Annabel was awarded an MBE ("Member of the British Empire") by the Queen, honoring her for her outstanding work in the field of child nutrition.

Her website www.annabelkarmel.com is one of the most popular sites for recipes and advice on feeding children.

Acknowlegments

Author's Acknowledgments
A big thank you to my wonderful team at DK: Peggy Vance, Helen Murray, Sara Kimmins, Charlotte Seymour, Penny Warren, Marianne Markham, Glenda Fisher, and Caroline Gibson. I also want to thank Dave King, Seiko Hatfield, Liz Thomas, Caroline Stearns, Marina Magpoc, Evelyn Etkind, and Tripp Trapp (for kindly loaning us their high chairs). A special thanks to all my gorgeous babies and their moms and dads.

Publisher's Acknowledgments
DK would like to thank Jo Godfrey Wood for editorial assistance, Sarah Ponder for initial design styling, Susan Bosanko for the index, Becky Alexander for proofreading, and Roisin Donaghy and Jo Penford for hair and makeup. DK would also like to thank all the models: Craig and Thomas Barrington; Susannah Blyth-Corcoran and Amélie Lecoeur; Sarah Booker and Ellie Walker; Noah Catchpole; Pinny and Kit Crane; Leigh and Isla Haynes; Nathalie and Charlie Heath; Emmanuelle and Joachim Horsford; Susanna and Poppy Howe; Vanessa Josephs and Caelan Edie; Susan Knox and Cormac Joseph Knox Heinrich; Suzanne and Sadie Lander; Lesley Manalo and Nathan De Castro; Esther Marney and Amelie Read; Daniel Pirrie; Viv and Aaron Ridgeway. All images © Dorling Kindersley